Anne Woodham is a highly r̶... ̶...̶g̶
mother. A former health ed... ̶a̶n̶d̶ deputy editor of *Good Housekeeping*, she succumbed to feeling Tired All The Time. She has now conquered her fatigue and writes the Mind and Body column for *Good Housekeeping*.

This is her story and much more besides as she shows the way, with humour and compassion, to stop feeling tired.

Jonathan Pugh is a highly successful cartoonist whose work appears regularly in the *Independent* and in the *Guardian* and *The Times*. He has illustrated a number of books.

GET UP AND GO!

Self help for
fatigue sufferers

Anne Woodham

HEADLINE

First published in 1994
by HEADLINE BOOK PUBLISHING

10 9 8 7 6 5 4 3 2 1

ISBN 0 7472 4335 2

Typeset by
Letterpart Limited, Reigate, Surrey

Printed and bound in Great Britain by
HarperCollins Manufacturing, Glasgow

HEADLINE BOOK PUBLISHING
A division of Hodder Headline PLC
Headline House
79 Great Titchfield Street
London W1P 7FN

To Stephen, Tamsin and Jonathan

Contents

1.	Tired all the time	1
2.	Is there a medical reason for your fatigue?	12
3.	The alternative route	39
4.	Is it really ME?	52
5.	Is your environment getting you down?	64
6.	Stressbusting	76
7.	What you can do immediately . . .	92
8.	Eating for energy	108
9.	Get fit to fight fatigue	128
10.	Take a good look at yourself	142
11.	Getting your act together	155
12.	Release your healing resources	171
13.	All in the mind	185
14.	Last but not least	206
	Index	210

CHAPTER 1

Tired all the time

TATT

'There's not really anything wrong with me. Nothing you could put your finger on. It's just that I feel so tired all the time.'

Tired All The Time. Doctors hear that phrase so often that it's referred to in the trade as the TATT syndrome, frequently (and unfairly) attached to what are called 'heartsink' patients – people whose mere appearance in the surgery makes the heart sink. Poor doctors, however. Many of them suffer from TATT themselves; they're worn out and impatient and somebody wittering about feeling tired doesn't exactly turn on their taps of loving kindness.

But there's a lot of TATT about. Business executives battling through twelve-hour days in the office; secretaries and stock-brokers hip to thigh in crowded peak hour trains; teachers burning the midnight oil over Form Five's history essays; sales reps; shop-owners; taxi drivers; editors and accountants. And working mothers – oh, especially working mothers: coming home to find the cat has been sick, the fridge is empty and 'I forgot to tell you, mum, but I need my costume for the school play by tomorrow.' There's instantaneous gold-plated exhaustion for you.

It comes as absolutely no surprise to learn that one third of women between 18 and 39 complain of 'always feeling tired', and the more young children they have, the worse they feel. Well, of course. Men are almost as bad. In the same report in the *British Medical Journal*, 20 per cent of men complained of persistent tiredness.

At least half the adult population of Great Britain will suffer from TATT at some time. That's a virtual epidemic. Unlike ME, the so-called 'yuppie flu', TATTers keep stumbling into work, though they feel lethargic and listless and have a hard time stifling their yawns.

Going to bed early doesn't help. In a recent study, 48 per cent of people said they still feel exhausted after a good night's sleep, and four out of ten of these said they felt that way every day.

Some people pick up in a few months, others totter along with TATT for years. Doctors can't put their finger on specific sources. One psychiatrist describes it as 'a medical mystery'. Stress, say some. Depression, claim others. A product of high-speed modern living, most agree.

Surprisingly few people consult their doctors, although GPs say persistent fatigue is one of the most common complaints they hear. One in every ten people in the doctor's surgery reports feeling tired all the time. And in another study – to give an inkling of the extent of the problem – for every woman who told her GP, another 400 confessed to bouts of fatigue.

TATT is no joke and shouldn't be dismissed. Treat it as a warning. This is not a disease but a *symptom* that something is wrong with us – physically, mentally, emotionally or spiritually. Its knock-on effect is enormous, even lethal. Tired people are cross, irritable people who pass on their disgruntlement to those around them. Mistakes are made, resentments fester. In about one third of sufferers the cause is an underlying physical problem that more often than not can be treated. And besides, in 90 per cent of cases of TATT, whatever the origin, Something Can Be Done. It's so easy to say change your way of looking at things, but it *can* help. Look at it not so much as 'I'm feeling tired and feeble', but 'how can I find more energy?' At least asking a question is action of a sort.

WORKING MUMS

'For the last twenty years I've been running with my head down, getting my career going, having kids, moving house, and

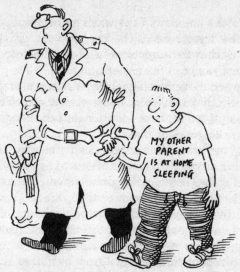

I'm very, very tired,' says Christine, communications director for a top advertising agency. Her husband is chief executive of another agency, and they have two children, aged ten and five.

'I've achieved a lot, but I'm not happy with the pace of my life. It's going too fast, and I feel as if I'm on a conveyor belt and want to jump off. I'm one of those women who tend to do too much and I know I haven't the energy I had at 25. You can get so bogged down by all the tedious things of running a household, and sometimes you get too finicky and pernickety about it all. And then you want to do the extras as well – decorating, gardening, exercising, entertaining. It's damn difficult to fit it all in.

'I can't keep going all day – I get tired, and I get PMT badly and I'm grumpy with the family. Every weekend I have a migraine or a backache and it's boring. You can't go on feeling knackered all your life.'

As far as most women are concerned, the New Man who shares the chores is a myth. It's mum who, even before her coat is off her back after work, has put the rice on for supper. She runs the children's baths, reads the bedtime book, helps with home-

3

work, loads the laundry in the washing machine, takes it out, puts it in the dryer, sweeps the kitchen floor, checks everyone has clean clothes for tomorrow, and topples into bed where, with any luck, she can fall asleep and not have to play at being Kim Basinger. Research supports this sorry state: working mothers average 36 hours on housework and childcare a week; their husbands watch television for an hour longer and sleep half an hour longer each night.

Working mothers talk about sleep the way that hungry people talk about food. When interviewed by American sociologist Dr Arlie Hochschild, they complained compulsively about being overtired, sick and 'emotionally drained'. They discussed how much sleep they could 'get by on' – six and a half hours, seven, seven and a half, less, more. Some apologised 'I'm afraid I need eight hours of sleep' as if eight hours were too much. They talked about how travel threw out sleep patterns, and how to avoid waking up completely when a child cried at night, and how to get back to sleep again. I remember being woken – barely two seconds after sinking stone-like into oblivion – by the whimper of a child winding itself up for a good yell, and willing it to 'Go To Sleeeeeep', as if the sheer force of my mental command would stun it into silence. Sometimes, astonishingly, it worked – but mostly not.

TECHNOLOGICAL TYRANNY

But one has to be fair. Working mothers don't have a monopoly on fatigue. The culture we live in has stratospheric expectations of its members; each new labour-saving invention only means time freed for yet more work. Once you could board a plane or train and read a book, blissfully secure in the knowledge that you were beyond reach of the office. Now you must open your lap top and flex your credit card for the inflight telephone.

A million years ago, it seems – before computers had found their way into every office and school and home – I interviewed a scientist who spoke dreamily of the brave new world ahead: hours of leisure at our disposal, he predicted, while computers despatched in moments the work that had taken human brains hours and days to achieve.

Boy, did he have it wrong! Somebody has to feed the machines their data, so faster and faster we go, producing facts and figures to keep the electronic tyrants busy. Reams of information and vast sums of money are transferred from one side of the world to the other in seconds, decisions taken, events shaped. A mere decade ago you wrote a letter and waited in a civilised way for the reply – three days, a week perhaps. Now you fax in the morning and act on the response in the afternoon.

In exactly the same way the vacuum cleaner was hailed as the housewife's great liberator – and what happened? Did women lie about eating chocolates and improving their minds with Proust? Not a bit of it. The hours spent in sweeping and beating were cleared for polishing and pickling, cooking and cleaning. Houses gleamed as never before, wonderful glass towers in which women found themselves imprisoned.

Now the office blocks are prisons too: the nine to five day stretches from eight to seven. Ashen-faced businessmen and women totter home with bulging briefcases of work to catch up on, papers to keep abreast of. Professional journals, 'must read' documents; never has there been such mountains of information, words and diagrams, charts and graphs, spewing out of laser printers and dancing across computer screens. Our poor brains are in overload.

So are our bodies. We invented aeroplanes so we have to throw ourselves around the world in them, knocking our biorhythms out of kilter. We arrive in London in the morning after a night flight from New York: the clock says eight, but our body says 4 a.m., when all our functions are at their lowest ebb.

Planes, trains, cars, computers, washing machines – they can all pound away twenty-four hours a day, but what about the poor humans who are supposed to control them? The 1990 Aerospace Medical Association Conference reported a commercial flight across the Pacific to Seattle. The plane ignored air traffic controllers' instructions to descend and flew on over Seattle airport, up into Canadian airspace, where interceptor jets from the Royal Canadian Airforce failed to make radio contact. In desperation they buzzed the airliner, flashing blinding lights into the cockpit. Finally the crew woke up, looked at each other in horror and turned the plane round.

Tired, you see. Worn out.

STRESS FALLOUT

Don't ignore persistent fatigue. It can be a warning that you are under too much stress for your own health's sake.

When we're tired we lose our sense of proportion. Our judgement is askew; everyday events take on a cataclysmic perspective. 'When I'm at the end of my tether, the children's rowing drives me over the edge,' said one mother, a teacher. 'Perfectly innocuous remarks, like "when's supper?" make me erupt. The house seems dirtier, the children scruffier, colleagues less caring. Nothing is possible, I'll never get my marking done, the students will fail their exams and it will all be my fault. Aaaargh.'

We all know there is fatigue and fatigue. There's the kind of honest muck and sweat fatigue, for instance, that comes after a long hard day of exertion. The end of a ten-mile rough country hike. A day spent moving furniture, or digging up the garden. Making jam, sewing curtains, running a jumble sale, writing an essay, polishing the car, playing tennis. That well-earned sense of physical and mental exhaustion in the evening as you slump in front of the television set, and finally, glowing with self-satisfaction, slide gratefully into bed.

But this book is about persistent fatigue, the Tired All The Time kind, when you wake up unrefreshed and the thought of a bright new day leaves you unmoved; the hours ahead like lumpen boulders to be pushed at and clambered over. When the thought of commuting and cleaning and shuffling papers and

6

picking up children is wearying beyond measure; when looking at teenagers' filthy, clothes-littered, cup-cluttered, mouldy crumb-scattered bedrooms makes you want to weep. When you feel that life is like lying under a pile of old overcoats from which it seems impossible to fight your way out.

This kind of fatigue can be a sympton of stress, when we're under too much pressure. A bit of stress, in fact, is no bad thing, otherwise we'd never get anything done at all. If I didn't have a deadline for this book, for instance, I wouldn't be pecking at the word processor when I could be lying in bed reading the Sunday papers. If you didn't have to keep a roof over your head and buy food, would you bother getting up and earning the wherewithal to do so? Without the stress of keeping off sabre-toothed tigers, would our cave-dwelling ancestors have got around to discovering fire?

Stress is a pretty individual thing. What is stressful for me might not be so for you. The thought of speaking in public

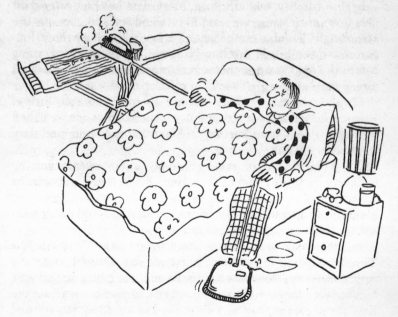

brings Nick out in a lather of perspiration – all those people looking at him: what if he stutters? What if he can't think what to say? – whereas Judy loves it. She knows she does it well and she can't wait for the moment when the audience's eyes are on her, laughing when she makes a joke, listening to her voice and what she has to say.

Jim is a solicitor, preparing briefs for court cases. He simply can't crank himself into action until the last possible moment. 'I have to reach the point when to leave things another day would be too late and I've frightened myself. Then I work twenty hours at a stretch, fuelled by coffee and adrenalin. It's agony at the time, but the buzz when I finish is fantastic.'

Margaret, on the other hand, loathes being rushed. Too much on her plate or last minute demands, and she feels panicky. 'I can't think straight,' she says. 'I don't know what to do first. I like everything organised, sorted out well in advance.'

In the ordinary way of things, most of us have a pretty good idea how much stress we can tolerate and try and pace our life accordingly. Trouble comes when we lose control of events, like surfers whose heads are barely above water after one wave before the next is upon them. Problems seem to come from all directions – at home, at work, in relationships – and the bigger the wave, the more likely we are to come up spluttering. Divorce, bereavement, redundancy – these are what we called dumpers when I went surfing in Australia as a child, and they can knock you out.

But a succession of even relatively minor events can be exhausting, if you don't have time to rest and recover in between.

Often it's a combination of the anticipated and the unexpected. You're a junior sales manager: you take out a mortgage for a new house, preparing yourself to be financially stretched for a period – but not for your partner's unplanned pregnancy, your mother to become seriously ill, and your boss to demand higher sales targets if the company is to survive lean times. You work longer hours, every weekend you drive a two-hundred-mile round trip to see your mother, you lie awake at night worrying about money and babies, sex is hardly worth the effort and you're grey with fatigue. You come down with a cold – stress dampens the immune system so you're more susceptible to passing viruses – and you get a parking ticket. Then your secretary botches up a letter for the third time and it's the last straw. You lose your rag and shout at her. So you feel mean, and angry with her for making you feel mean. She complains, your boss lectures you about staff relations, and on we go . . . The stress-fatigue-stress cycle is nicely established.

In theory, with enough sleep, adequate exercise and good nutrition (*not* skipping breakfast and snacking on a Crunchie bar and coffee for lunch), we should have enough energy to cope – and if not, then it's probably wise to examine your way of life. Be honest and ask yourself a few straight questions. This is not the moment for self-delusion.

★ Will the pressures be short-term?
★ Are you in the right kind of job?
★ Do you organise your time as well as you could?
★ Are there activities and commitments you could cut out or postpone?
★ Do you share problems with those who care about you?
★ Do you 'reward' yourself enough? A night out having a good laugh with friends isn't just an indulgence: American research shows that in lonely people, without family or friends to fall back on, the body's natural killer cells that fight off disease are suppressed.

IS IT A SYMPTOM OF DISEASE?

Stress-induced or not, fatigue should always be taken seriously. At least a third of patients in the doctor's surgery complaining of TATT turn out to have a genuine medical reason for their persistent fatigue.

'Of course I'm tired,' I used to say as I pinched myself to keep awake at friends' dinner parties. 'I've got two children and a job and a basket of ironing.'

'If only I could take a holiday,' I puffed after climbing two flights of stairs at the office. My head spun like a fairground razzledazzle. 'Thank God tomorrow's Saturday. If I get to the supermarket in the morning maybe I can snatch a nap after lunch.'

I saw the doctor for a repeat prescription for the Pill. 'Routine visit,' I assured her. 'There's nothing wrong with me. Just too much work.'

'Rubbish,' she said, examining my hand. 'Look at your fingernails. They're too pale. We're taking a blood sample right now. My guess is you've got anaemia.'

She was right.

A course of iron tablets and I felt a new woman. But how did things get to such a pass? I'd suffered heavy periods for months but never got round to doing anything about them – too busy, reluctant to make a fuss, just something else to put up with. And anyway, if you have a full-time job and a family, I convinced myself, fatigue is part of the furniture.

But why should it be? Fatigue – the relentless, debilitating exhaustion that so many people complain of – shouldn't be normal. Whatever the cause, there's no reason to lie back and accept it. If a medical condition is responsible, then it's vital to make a diagnosis and start treatment. Often there are complementary therapies, too, which can work hand in hand with modern drugs and surgery.

Maybe the root of the fatigue is even deeper and more complicated. Depression, grief, anger, anxiety, loneliness and boredom – these are feelings we often try to ignore because they seem too big and scary to confront. We squash them away and then, like an overstuffed suitcase, they burst the locks and spill out over the corners.

Some people don't even *know* they're tired,' says Jane McWhirter of All Hallows House, an alternative health centre in the City of London which unravels exhausted and knotted financiers. 'They keep going so hard they don't allow themselves time to think.'

Our poor immune systems take such a battering that we succumb, in the end, to any manner of conditions. Chronic fatigue syndrome is one; a ghastly spiral where fatigue leads to depression to fatigue to depression to . . . Then all the foundations of our life must be examined and re-built, a painful and revolutionary experience.

And yet sometimes a little common sense doesn't go astray. Karen, a young single mother with a new baby, was exhausted. The baby cried, she cried, her tiny flat was dirty, and there never seemed time or energy to tidy up, or get herself dressed properly. The doctor talked gravely about post-natal depression, fostering and antidepressants; the health visitor, who was a practical and perceptive woman, arranged for someone to clean the flat and mind the baby while Karen went to the hairdresser and met friends. It wasn't a lot, a couple of hours a week, but it tipped the balance. Karen still got tired, the way all new mothers get tired, but the baby gurgled and there was light at the end of the tunnel.

Reference

The Second Shift by Dr Arlie Hochschild (Piatkus)

CHAPTER 2

Is there a medical reason for your fatigue?

DOCTOR'S ORDERS

So you're exhausted. You even wake up feeling tired. A couple of good nights' sleep or a holiday hasn't improved matters, and you can't find any obvious reasons – such as a new baby or new job – for feeling like an old dish mop that's done a plate too many. Drag yourself together and totter along to your GP. In at least a third of people who complain of persistent fatigue, the cause is physical.

Steel yourself for an initial glazing over of the eyes by His Medicalness. Chances are you're the umpteenth person in the surgery that week to complain of feeling 'tired all the time'. The doctor is probably feeling pretty shattered himself – spare a thought for him: a surgery full of coughs and colds, endless NHS paperwork, referrals to write, housecalls to make, sad news to break to a terminally ill patient, and you're sitting there saying wimpy things like 'well, there's nothing particularly wrong with me, it's just that I seem to be always so tired'.

But don't let your sympathy – or the doctor's dismissiveness – prevent you from standing your ground. You know your fatigue is real and it's interfering with your life enough to get you down to the surgery, so make sure you state your case – exhausting though it may be.

If you're the kind of person who's easily flummoxed when talking to doctors (and that's most of us, if truth be known) write what you want to say on a piece of paper and take it with

What to tell the doctor

It helps to think through your answers to the following questions. And if the doctor doesn't ask them, that doesn't stop you supplying the information.

★ How long have you been feeling tired?
★ Do you feel tired even after a good night's sleep or a relaxing weekend?
★ How much does it affect your way of life? Are you too exhausted to make love, for instance? To go out with friends or take gentle exercise?
★ Are there other symptoms – such as an allergy, loss of appetite, cough, thirst, sweats, irritability, pain, muscle weakness, change in bladder or bowel habits?
★ If you are a woman, are your periods heavier or lighter than usual? Could you be approaching the menopause?
★ Do you have (or have you had) an infection or illness?
★ Are you losing weight?
★ Have you had a recent emotional shock, such as a bereavement, divorce or redundancy?
★ Did the fatigue come on suddenly, or did it creep up on you?
★ Do you feel tired at a certain time of the day or week (Monday morning, for example) or year?
★ Is it worse in certain kinds of weather?
★ Do you have trouble sleeping?
★ Are you taking any prescribed drugs or any medical treatment?
★ Is your fatigue worse when you're in a particular building or place, or when with certain people?
★ Have you changed your eating habits? Gone on a diet, perhaps?
★ How often do you exercise?
★ Do you smoke or drink alcohol, tea or coffee? How much?
★ Have you travelled abroad recently?

you. You might feel a prat pulling it out, but better that than come away kicking yourself for forgetting something vital. Doctors are only human – especially if they're in a hurry and you're fumbling and mumbling.

But do remember this: **persistent and inexplicable fatigue can be one of several symptoms for a number of medical conditions, some of them serious.** The fact that you get dizzy when you stand up suddenly or climb stairs, or that you're always thirsty or peeing more than usual *as well as feeling tired* are actually important things to get across, no matter how crabby and impatient your GP.

Do I have to see the doctor?
Yes. It's essential for the doctor to make a diagnosis. Orthodox medicine has an armoury of efficient treatments for the more common physical complaints of which fatigue is a symptom. And remember that fatigue is always a *symptom* of a malaise, whether physical, mental or emotional – not the disease itself.

MEDICAL REASONS FOR FEELING TIRED

1. Allergy
Bother lambs and blossom – in spring I'm so weary I toddle off to bed after supper. My eyes itch, I have violent and uncontrollable bouts of sneezing and a continual snuffle, and I am vile to know. Yes, it's hayfever. The pollen and grass seeds in the air at this time of year irritate the lining of my nose and throat, and I feel bunged up, lethargic, depressed, and very tired.

Hayfever is one of many allergies that can leave you feeling as if a vacuum cleaner has sucked out all your stuffing. What is an allergy? It's an abnormal sensitivity to particular foods, plants, animals, or insect bites, that triggers a physical reaction. Fatigue is a common response because the body's systems are under strain. Others might be migraine, eczema, rashes, nausea, diarrhoea, asthma or sneezing. If you're suffering from any of these, as well as feeling tired, an allergy could be the culprit.

What happens is that your body's immune system – your defence against disease – starts behaving like Arnold Schwarzenegger's Terminator. It becomes confused and mistakes harmless substances, such as pollen, dust or wheat, for dangerous invaders. Breathing or touching even the tiniest amounts of the **allergen** (the substance you are sensitive to) puts your defences on red alert. Protein substances called **antibodies** are released ready for battle. When they encounter the allergens, more chemicals called **histamines** are released, and it's these that are responsible for the actual allergic reaction.

Seemingly innocuous things can suddenly provoke physical uproar for no apparent reason. Animal hair, feathers, plants, soap, and cosmetics that you got along with very nicely thank you may turn round and cause mayhem. Even food: milk and dairy products, nuts, shellfish, fish, wheat and flour, chocolate and artificial colourings are notorious villains.

Sometimes it's hard to make a link, especially with certain foods. The reaction is slow – i.e. you don't vomit or collapse with exhaustion instantaneously – and the food (or additive) responsible is usually eaten frequently: wheat and milk, for example, pop up at most meals disguised in bread and tea.

A bad bout of flu or diarrhoea can spark a food intolerance, but mostly it sneaks up on you. Unlike serious food allergies which can last a lifetime, a food *intolerance* may disappear if the food can be identified and avoided for a few months.

'I'd been under a lot of stress – a friend had died after a long illness and we'd moved house – and I couldn't seem to pick myself up,' says Charlotte, a freelance film producer in her late thirties. 'I had this terrible fatigue – I felt absolutely leaden, as if I was swamped under an eiderdown, and my mind seemed incredibly thick. I couldn't work, because my brain felt like a television set where the circuits are fuzzy and everything is askew. I was so tired that I'd spend all weekend in bed and yet it wouldn't make any difference.

'At the same time I had this appalling depression, utterly suicidal, there was no point to anything in life at all, and I also developed this weird thing about eating, mindless munching all the time. Everything I ever suffered from got worse – terrible PMT, awful aches and pains in my fingers. I saw my GP, even a shrink, but they couldn't help my fatigue and depression. Increasingly I had a gut instinct that the cause lay in my diet.

'Finally I went to an alternative health practitioner, who did homeopathy, aromatherapy, reflexology – and dowsing. She got out her pendulum and ran it over my body and said, "Do you eat bread and pasta?"

' "All the time," I said. "Toast for breakfast, sandwiches for lunch and pasta for supper." '

' "Give wheat products a miss for 48 hours," she advised. I did, and in 24 hours I was a different person, and a week later I felt wonderful. I've kept off wheat ever since and I'm full of bounce again. I might eat the odd slice of bread, though I try and buy loaves made from untreated wheat flour at healthfood shops, and occasionally pasta if nothing else is available, but if I do I sense that lowness coming back, the beginnings of the old symptoms.'

Self-help
a) Identify the allergen if possible
Easier said than done. Take hayfever again, one of the most common allergies. In spring and summer about one in five people function on half cylinders because there's a lot of pollen about. But *what kind of pollen*? Tree pollen? Grass pollen? Or plant pollen? And if it's tree pollen, which tree? Ash? Hawthorn? Privet?

There are a couple of allergy tests you can take. One is a simple skin prick test, in which the suspect is applied to a patch of scratched skin and you wait for it to go red and come up in a lump. The second is more complicated and expensive and

16

involves sending a blood sample to a laboratory, but is also more precise.

A food intolerance might need an elimination diet to flush it out. This is best done under supervision – a doctor, naturopath or clinical ecologist – though if you suspect that a single food, such as chocolate or eggs, is causing your problem, try avoiding it for a week or two, and see what happens. Never cut out more than one food at a time.

b) Avoid it
Again often easier said than done. However, you can do the following:

★ Check food labels, if you suspect food additives. Eat fresh, unprocessed and organic foods.
★ Take care with household products. Wear rubber gloves.
★ Vacuum often – i.e. daily – if you think dust mites or animal hairs are the problem. This is a real pain when you're feeling tired, but could be worth the effort. Be warned: ordinary vacuums can make the situation worse by mixing allergens in the air, but some vacuum cleaners such as Medivac and Miele have special filters.
★ Stay indoors if you suffer from hayfever.

c) Treat the symptoms
According to your allergy, the doctor may prescribe antihistamines, cortisone sprays and creams, nose drops or bronchodilators. They work, on the whole, but some can have side effects like drowsiness – just what you need when you're already suffering from fatigue. Ask if there's an alternative, or hope that the treatment works fast.

Hayfever sufferers can buy a number of over-the-counter homeopathic remedies in health shops, but these can be rather hit and miss. A homeopath prescribes remedies tailored to the individual's personality and her specific symptoms; over-the-counter products often contain a range of substances in the hope that everyone will find something that works for them.

References

The National Society for Research into Allergy,
  PO Box 45,
  Hinckley,
  Leics. LE10 1JY
  (send large s.a.e.)
  (tel. 0455 851546)

Action Against Allergy,
  24-26 High Street,
  Hampton Hill,
  Middlesex TW12 1PD
  (send s.a.e.)

2. Anaemia

Blood ferries oxygen to every part of the body, where it powers the various organs and muscles. If your blood doesn't contain enough haemoglobin (the substance that carries oxygen) then imagine how you'll feel: tired, irritable, dizzy, short of breath, headachey and bone-achey and prone to every bug going around. You might also have swollen ankles, brittle or concave fingernails, a sore tongue, heart palpitations, problems with vision, loss of appetite and insomnia, and the occasional fainting fit. You'll probably look pale and less than interesting – a great test is the colour of your fingernails and the inner lining of your eyelids. In short, you'll be anaemic.

There are four main types of anaemia, and it's important that your doctor diagnoses which one you're suffering from.

a) Iron deficiency

Iron deficiency is the most common, and the reason that so many women complain of TATT. Thirty per cent of females between 30 and 40 suffer from it, and over an average lifetime, women need twice as much iron as men.

Women are great at worrying over their partners and kids

and force-feeding them steaks and broccoli and slabs of wholemeal bread, but we can be appalling at looking after ourselves. Test yourself: you're dishing out supper. Who gets the biggest helping? Your husband? Your teenage son or daughter? Chances are it won't be you – and yet you're probably the one in the family most in need of iron-rich meat and green veg.

Every cell in the body needs iron to do its job, and haemoglobin is stuffed with it (as well as oxygen). Women lose iron when they lose blood. This can be during childbirth, miscarriage, abortion, or surgery for fibroids, and – by far and away the most common – through heavy menstrual periods.

With the latter, you can slide into anaemia without realising it's even happening. Because the body stores iron in the liver, spleen, bone marrow and other tissues, it can take months and even years for stocks to run low.

My periods were horrendously heavy, but I was so concerned about how to deal with the flow and whether I had enough sanitary towels for emergencies that when each month was over I put the whole subject behind me until next time. I thought I ate reasonably well – what I didn't appreciate was that I should be eating *more* of the right kind of foods. I was working hard, so I put my fatigue down to stress, and spent most Saturday and Sunday afternoons lying on my bed resting. Until I happened to go to the doctor for an altogether different reason, and she – shrewd woman – said, 'Excuse me, but I think you might be anaemic.'

b) Pernicious anaemia

Pernicious anaemia is found in people who don't get enough vitamin B12. This is necessary to make blood and comes in animal products, so vegetarians and vegans – who eat no meat or dairy products – should take steps to compensate. Some people need monthly injections of vitamin B12 because they lack a stomach enzyme called, mysteriously, 'the intrinsic factor', which the body needs to absorb it. This is a type of megaloblastic anaemia.

c) Megaloblastic anaemia

Megaloblastic anaemia is caused by a shortage of folic acid, one of the B vitamins. Women who are pregnant, who have a lot of children, take oral contraceptives and/or are malnourished should watch their diet and take vitamin supplements if necessary. Serious dieters who cut nutritional corners can find themselves in the same boat.

d) Sickle-cell anaemia and thalassemia

Sickle-cell anaemia and thalassemia are inherited forms of anaemia which mainly affect African and Caribbean people (sickle-cell anaemia) and those from the Mediterranean and Asia (thalassemia).

Self-help

If you're low in iron, the best way to get enough is through your diet. Good sources are as follows:

★ Lean red meats, rich in the most easily absorbed form of iron. Liver is terrific, but it's also high in cholesterol so shouldn't be eaten more than once a week.

★ Chicken and fish, which contain one third to one half the iron in red meat. About 15–30 per cent of iron in meat, fish and poultry is absorbed by the body, compared to an average 5 per cent from vegetables, fruit, grains and eggs.

★ Peas, beans, corn.

★ Bread, cereals or pasta labelled 'enriched' or 'fortified'. Wholemeal bread can actually 'bind' iron, limiting its absorption.

★ Foods high in vitamin C, because they help the body absorb iron: citrus fruits and juices, tomatoes, sweet peppers, broccoli, cauliflower, leafy greens, strawberries and potatoes with skin. Popeye was on to a bit of a bummer with spinach though – its high oxalic acid content slows iron absorption.

★ Combinations of vegetables, fruit and grain with meat and fish for maximum absorption. Try chili con carne: chili beans and lean minced beef or lamb pack a double punch. The vitamin

20

C in orange juice is brilliant; drink with a vegetarian meal – or
any sort of meal – to enhance your iron intake.
★ Iron cooking pots – the iron seeps into the food.

If you're still worried about whether your intake is adequate, iron
supplements might be a good idea, but for heaven's sake consult
your doctor. Iron pills are also notorious for causing constipation
and dark, tarry stools, which can be somewhat disconcerting.
(Check *any* dark stools with your GP; see **Cancer** below.)
 There are no 'alternative' cures for anaemia, but the following could be tried as complementary therapy, with your GP's
approval:

Homeopathic remedies
(These are available in health-food shops): ferrum; natrum
mur.; china for blood loss and exhaustion; picric for anaemia
coupled with mental overload; arsenicum for pernicious
anaemia; calcarea phos. for children and adolescents.

Aromatherapy
Add ten drops each of the essential oils of Roman camomile and
lemon each to 50 ml. of vegetable oil and rub into your body
after a bath or shower.

Herbal medicine
Infusions of angelica, centaury or wild chicory leaves, horsetail,
nettle, rosemary flowers or leaves, strawberry and thyme.
(Check with a medical herbalist if you think you might be
pregnant.)

3. Cancer
Persistent tiredness for no apparent reason can be a symptom
of cancer – which is why you should see the doctor *at once* if you
also have any of the following:

★ Weight loss that you can't explain.
★ Indigestion for no particular reason.

★ Blood in your urine or faeces, whether red or dark and tarry.

★ Changes in your bowel habits; diarrhoea or constipation lasting more than two weeks.

★ Constant coughing and/or spitting up blood.

★ Ulcers and skin sores that refuse to heal.

★ Moles that change shape or colour, become itchy or bleed.

★ Any inexplicable lumps, especially in the breast, neck or testicles.

★ Puckering or unusual changes in the shape of the breasts.

★ Any vaginal bleeding or blood-stained discharge between periods, after sex or after the menopause.

4. Candida albicans (Thrush)

We share our bodies with a yeast-like fungal organism called monilia or candida albicans. It likes warm moist places and can be found in the mouth, bowel, vagina, and on the vulva and skin. Mostly it quietly minds its own business, but occasionally it goes bananas, growing rampageously, weakening the immune system that fights disease and triggering an infection known as *thrush*.

This causes sore white patches on the skin, or if in the vagina, itchiness and a thick curdy white discharge that smells like baking bread. Fat people can develop it in the folds of their skin, and people whose hands are in water a lot may find a little infection doing very nicely thank you under their fingernails. It's accompanied by fatigue and a general 'blah' feeling, often noticed before the thrush appears. Lethargy, depression, headaches, bloatedness, allergies, cystitis and pre-menstrual tension have also been associated with candida infection.

Candida thrives on sugar, and is a particular problem for diabetics, whose blood and urine have excess sugar. Other people prone to thrush are pregnant women, in whom the cells lining the vagina have a high glycogen content; the very young and the very old; those debilitated by leukaemia, cancer and AIDS; people with iron deficiency anaemia (the only time I got thrush was when I was anaemic); those taking steroids and the oral contraceptive

Pill, and anyone on antibiotics – these kill off the friendly bacteria which normally keep candida under control.

The doctor may take a swab to confirm the presence of candida, or test for diabetes. Effective drugs prescribed are nystatin, clotrimazole (Canesten) or imidazole. There are a number of homeopathic remedies but you really need to see a homeopath for an expert diagnosis.

Self-help
a) Oral thrush

★ Aloe vera mouthwash (available from chemists and health-food stores) is an antifungal agent.
★ Gargle with three drops of tea tree essential oil and one drop of essential oil of myrrh in half a glass of water.
★ Tinctures of myrrh or marigold are recommended herbal mouthwashes.

b) Vaginal thrush

★ Wear cotton underwear and change daily.
★ Avoid tights, wear stockings or socks instead.
★ Don't use vaginal deodorants, perfumed bath oils, soaps, or talcum powder.
★ Don't wash your clothes in strong detergent.
★ Wear a sanitary pad and not a tampon during menstruation.
★ Exercise regularly and avoid constipation.
★ Wash with a solution of one tablespoon of salt to one pint of water.
★ Acidophilus and live bio-yoghurt replace the 'good' bacteria which keeps candida albicans under control. Take by mouth or as a vaginal douche. Spread live yoghurt on a sanitary towel or tampon for easier application.

In general:

★ Cut all sugars, even honey, from your diet.

★ Avoid alcohol, tea, coffee and chocolate.
★ Avoid carbohydrates or any yeast products.
★ Take garlic, an antifungal agent, in capsule form.
★ Eat plenty of fresh vegetables, whole grains, beans of all kinds, and pumpkin, sesame and sunflower seeds.
★ Supplement your diet with vitamins C and B, zinc, and evening primrose oil.

5. Diabetes
Make sure you tell your doctor if you are suffering from the following:

★ Feeling increasingly weak and tired AND losing weight.
★ Thirsty all the time.
★ Peeing more than usual.
★ Suffering from itching genitals.

These are the symptoms of diabetes mellitus, which can happen suddenly and at any age. In normal circumstances the carbohydrate we eat as sugars and starches is broken down into glucose in the small intestine and enters the bloodstream. Here it meets insulin, a hormone secreted by cells in the pancreas, which helps it enter the body's cells to provide energy.

In a diabetic, the pancreas either fails to produce insulin (insulin-dependent diabetes mellitus) or the body cells won't respond to it. Regular insulin injections are often necessary and you must get adequate medical supervision.

'I took to dropping off in the bath at night,' says Nicola, the mother of two teenagers who is taking a university degree as a mature student. She discovered she had diabetes when she woke up from a coma in an ambulance speeding her to hospital. 'It was a bit scary – one night I got into the bath about midnight and woke up three hours later, feeling cold and quite awful. My husband had fallen asleep. It alarmed us both. I could have died of hypothermia or drowned, I suppose.

'The mental tiredness was the first indication that something might be wrong. I kept falling asleep all the time, in the afternoon after lunch, or in the early evening after supper, when my blood sugar levels would rise. I couldn't keep my eyes open during lectures or in conversations. It was agony, not being able to concentrate and not knowing whether I should be answering yes or no to people's questions.

'I suspected something was wrong – I was always thirsty and I was losing weight. This seemed so brilliant that I put off going to the doctor for far too long.'

Self-help
There's really nothing in the way of self-help for diabetics – you must see your GP without delay for treatment; but complementary therapists offer a few suggestions that might help balance the pancreas as much as possible:

★ Keep to a low-fat, low-salt, high-fibre diet, with whole grains, lentils, beans and vegetables such as spinach and jacket potatoes. Avoid refined carbohydrate such as white bread and sugar.
★ Herbalists recommend raw garlic to stop the increase of blood sugar.
★ Supplements of chromium, vitamins C and E and evening primrose oil may be useful, but consult a naturopath or nutrition therapist.
★ An aromatherapy bath oil of 6–8 drops each of camphor, eucalyptus, geranium, juniper, lemon and rosemary could help pancreatic functioning.
★ Hatha yoga could help balance body functions.

6. Hypoglycaemia
Strictly speaking, this is a diabetic condition known as 'going hypo', when there is too much insulin and too little glucose in the blood. The symptoms are weakness, hunger, nausea, sweating, trembling, mental confusion, irritability, emotional instability, slurred speech and ultimately coma. To prevent them being picked up as drunk and thrown into gaol while 'hypo',

many diabetics wear ID cards or bracelets to alert anyone finding them in this condition.

Non-diabetics may sometimes experience similar symptoms – extreme fatigue, panic attacks, palpitations, depression and hyperventilation or over-breathing. Hypoglycaemia! they cry. But – despite a lot of fashionable talk about high blood sugar levels – this is rarely due to a genuine glucose imbalance, but to excessive adrenalin generated by anxiety and made worse by an inadequate diet. Eating usually relieves the problem.

If you're prone to such attacks it might be sensible to eat regular small meals – four or five daily rather than three larger ones – and avoid stimulants such as tea and coffee. Make sure your diet is not overwhelmed by sugary and starchy foods: snack on fruit and not chocolate bars. See Chapter 8 for nutritional advice and Chapter 6 on how to cope with stress.

7. Menopause

Some women sail through the change of life hardly turning a hair. Lady Antonia Fraser, now 60, looks almost ten years younger; her periods stopped at 49, with no more ruffling of life's waters than 'a slight tendency to open the windows for fresh air'. Others go through hell: hot flushes, suicidal depression, sleepless nights drenched in sweat, dizziness, irrational mood swings, an inability to concentrate. Gail Sheehy, the American author of *The Silent Passage*, the recent bestseller on the menopause, describes 'little crashes of fatigue':

'Having always counted on abundant energy, it was profoundly upsetting to find myself sometimes crawling home from a day of writing and falling into bed for a "nap", from which I had to drag myself up just to have dinner.'

As in pregnancy, fatigue during the menopause can be monumental – but not every woman will be stricken by it. Our experiences of the great female milestones are uniquely individual, and yet equally valid. One girl's periods start at 11, another's at 15. I spent both my pregnancies in a blur of fatigue, my best friend was buzzing about until the day she went into labour. Antonia Fraser forged on regardless, Gail Sheehy collapsed in a heap.

Like pregnancy too, the menopause is not an illness, but it represents such an enormous turning point for women that sometimes it can be difficult to tease psychological and psychosomatic factors from the purely physical. It is not just the cessation of monthly periods, but the end of fertility. Old age knocks at the door. In a culture where mothers are valued for their ability to bear children, and women for their youth and beauty, a woman who is losing both may feel bereft of any usefulness or purpose in living.

How many of her menopausal problems – her lethargy and depression perhaps – stem from this crisis of identity and sense of mortality is not easy to judge. Is forgetfulness and fatigue merely a sign of ageing? And when the biochemical pathways of the psyche and the body are proving so inextricably related, how can we say that one symptom is 'all in the mind' and another 'physiologically valid'?

The term menopause covers that period when a woman stops menstruating and her fertility declines. This can be any time from the early forties to the mid fifties, and usually lasts two to three

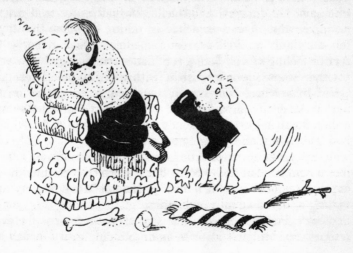

years, but may be longer. Gail Sheehy talks of a perimenopause that may begin eight years or more before periods cease.

But the bald facts are these: the ovaries stop producing eggs and production of the female hormone oestrogen diminishes. Physical results are as follows:

★ Menstrual changes: periods are skipped, scanty or flood so heavily you risk anaemia.
★ Hormonal fluctuations, which cause the infamous hot flushes and night sweating.
★ The vagina loses its lubricating fluid and becomes dry: sex seems less attractive.

A more ominous side effect of reduced oestrogen is the loss of bone mass that can result in **osteoporosis** and an increased risk of bone fractures.

Self-help
The most dramatic and controversial treatment is **HRT – hormone replacement therapy.** Some users swear it is the elixir of life. MP Teresa Gorman, a founder of the Amarant Trust which promotes HRT, has all the ardour of the convert. She says her fatigue, hot flushes, forgetfulness and apathy disappeared as soon as she started taking hormone therapy. 'I felt absolutely marvellous, restored, almost resurrected, with a terrific feeling of well-being, confidence and energy.'

Other women won't touch it with a barge pole. Germaine Greer in her book *The Change* suspects a conspiracy on the part of the drug companies, and claims postmenopausal women regain a new lease of confidence and energy naturally.

'I tried HRT and got migraine headaches,' says Gabrielle, who now visits an acupuncturist with, she claims, some allevia-tion of the sudden and violent hot flushes that drained her of energy and make her life a misery. She has taken to carrying a fan in her handbag as a precaution.

'I don't like the idea of taking synthetic hormones for ever,' worries Jane. 'I don't want to go on bleeding every month just when I thought I'd finished with tampons and sanitary pads, and I don't believe the jury is in yet on long-term risks of cancer.'

She is justified in thinking twice about HRT. Early research showed an increased risk of cancer of the womb lining from the oestrogen in HRT, but this is now offset by prescribing a parallel course of progestogen. Studies still show that after six years of taking HRT there is a small but undeniably increased risk of breast cancer. Further long-term research is now under way, but meanwhile millions of women are taking HRT in what American public health expert Dr Lewis Kuller calls 'the largest uncontrolled clinical trial in the history of medicine'.

But the advantages are enormous. Maintaining oestrogen levels with HRT unquestionably protects against osteoporosis, and reduces the risk of heart disease for women that rises after the menopause.

Each woman must make her own choice. How intolerable are her symptoms? Does she have a family history of cancer? Or of osteoporosis? What does seem clear is that if you can approach the menopause in a positive frame of mind, regarding it as an opportunity for freedom, fresh zest and new experiences, you'll reap benefits in the years ahead.

This may sound fanciful to someone who's struggling to get through the day without (a) spontaneously combusting; (b) screaming at their partner/child/boss/best friend/cat; or (c) crying 'goodbye cruel world forever' – but there are any number of **stress-reducing, coping and energising techniques,** for which see Chapters 6, 7 and 12. Try to get your mind off yourself if you can. It's also worth remembering that women busy in paid or voluntary work do seem to suffer less menopausal side effects.

For those who don't want or can't take HRT (it's not recommended for anyone with a history of cancer, for example), **other orthodox and complementary treatments** are available for menopausal symptoms. Homeopaths have a string of remedies at hand, but like to tailor them to individuals.

★ Good sex (*not* when you've just collapsed into bed for the night perhaps) can alleviate fatigue: it stimulates blood circulation, revs up the hormones and makes you feel 'stroked' and attractive. The GP may prescribe an oestrogen cream for vaginal dryness. Otherwise Replens and the good old standby KY Jelly are available over the counter.

★ Camomile tea and lime blossom tea can help you relax.

★ Add oats to your diet as a tonic.

★ Add six to eight drops of essential oils of sage, cypress and geranium to your bath to ease physical symptoms.

★ Homeopathic remedies lachesis and natrum mur. could help fatigue and irritability.

★ Make sure your diet is high in vitamins B, C, E and calcium, zinc and magnesium and, if necessary, take daily supplements.

★ Eat well, exercise and get enough sleep – but more, much more, on this later.

References

The Prime of Your Life by Pamela Armstrong (Headline)
The Silent Passage by Gail Sheehy (HarperCollins)
The Change by Germaine Greer (Hamish Hamilton)
Time of her Life by Dr Myra Hunter and Dr Jean Coope (BBC Books)
The Menopause: Coping with the Change by Dr Jean Coope (Optima)

The Amarant Trust
  80 Lambeth Road,
  London SE1 7PW
  (tel. 071-401 3855)
  Information on HRT and advice on midlife issues

National Osteoporosis Society,
  PO Box 10,
  Radstock,
  Bath,
  Avon BA3 3YB
  (tel. 0761 432472)

Menopause Clinics: check with your local Well Woman Clinic, Family Planning Clinic or gynaecology department of your local hospital, or contact the Amarant Trust.

8. Pain

Chronic pain is no joke, whatever the cause. It saps your strength and energy and even your will to live. At night you can't sleep and then, during the day, your fatigue makes the pain worse, and there seems to be no end to the cycle. Take a crumb of comfort from the fact that you're not alone. Back pain, the most common source of agony, has doubled in each of the past two decades and now grips 15 per cent of adults in any fortnight.

Assuming you have seen the doctor and nothing further can be done to alleviate the root cause of the pain, you must look at ways of treating the pain itself. Researchers like to measure pain in 'ouches'; how can we close the pain tolerance gateway so that fewer 'ouches' slip through to the brain?

Painkillers

These are available, but some people find them ineffective or are reluctant to accept side effects such as nausea and diarrhoea. A number of complementary therapies offer pain-relief techniques: osteopathy, hypnotherapy, biofeedback, autogenic training, psychotherapy, healing, homeopathy and yoga, for instance. In a recent study, back-pain patients at Kingston Hospital found that the Alexander Technique, which encourages better posture, enabled them to take up tennis and cycling again.

Acupuncture

This has proved especially successful for all kinds of pain, from backache to migraine – so much so it's not unusual to find pain-relief clinics and physiotherapy departments offering acupuncture – though not always on the NHS. Because they are looking at the patient as a whole, and not just the symptoms, acupuncturists ask a lot of questions about the nature of the pain. (See Chapter 3.) Is it worse in the cold, heat, damp or wind? Does it feel sharp, throbbing or burning? Where, they want to know, is the *Qi* (life energy) weak? Faced with the unpalatable fact that acupuncture works, Western doctors console themselves with scientific explanations: stimulating nerves can block pain signals to the brain; acupuncture points can release endorphins, natural pain-relieving substances.

Visualisation
Visualisation – using the imagination to picture your pain disappearing – has a particularly good track record, and is used by many of the pain clinics attached to some hospitals. One woman pictured her pain as a glacier melting under the sun.

It's one of the techniques used at Input, the pioneering holistic pain clinic at St Thomas's Hospital, London, where desperate sufferers learn to throw away their drugs and walking sticks in a four-week in-patient regime. They come to 'accept' that, although no one may wave a magic wand to make their pain go away, they can function around it.

Our feelings of pain stem as much from our minds as our bodies, says Dr Charles Pither, the consultant anaesthetist in charge of Input. Childhood, education, relationships, our job and our genes can influence our 'ouch' tolerance as much as our nerve endings. The Input regime involves **relaxation and sleep techniques; physical exercise** to stimulate the endorphins (rest can be the worst thing for pain); and a programme to encourage **positive attitudes** about yourself – not the 'I can't do the shopping so I'm a failure and a waste of space' line of thought.

Waiting lists are long for Input, but for information about similar programmes contact Ship (Self-Help Pain Management).

Coping With Pain, an audio tape which gives advice about coping with pain and a relaxation programme, is available from the Pain Relief Foundation.

References
Pain Relief Foundation,
  Rice Lane,
  Liverpool L9 1AE
  (tel. 051-523 1486)

Ship (Self-Help Pain Management),
  33 Kingsdown Park,
  Tankerton,
  Kent CT5 2DT
  (tel. 0227 264677 Ship Helpline)

9. Premenstrual Syndrome (PMT)

'The week before my period is due I can hardly drag myself about,' says Judy. 'I'm so tired I go to bed after supper and I feel awful – depressed, what's-the-point-of-living, utter hopelessness – and I wake up to the same grey grunge. It doesn't matter whether I've had to rush about or had a quiet day at home, I still feel exhausted, drained and irritable. I hate myself, and everyone hates me. And then the day my period starts, I wake up and it's a new world. Wonderful. It's almost worth the PMT for the joy of it lifting.'

Marian sees it differently: 'I'm not so much depressed as lethargic. Everything is too much effort – I just can't be bothered. I've even put off dinner parties the weekend before my period starts because I can't face the shopping and cooking.'

Fatigue is a classic symptom of premenstrual tension – along with mood swings, fluid retention, bloatedness, crabbiness, clumsiness ('oops, another cup gone . . . you really shouldn't let me wash up at this time of month') and a lack of sexual ardour. In fact, one can't but harbour a teensy, unworthy suspicion that *some* women will pass off any sort of bad behaviour as PMT. 'Sorry, hope you didn't mind me falling asleep during your presentation and then saying it was a lot of crap anyway, but it's the old PMT.'

There's an argument that PMT doesn't exist, that it's all in the mind of women wanting to attract attention, and another that 90 per cent are crippled by it to such an extent they should avoid driving, crucial meetings and wearing black. (Better not breathe, either.) The truth, as always, is probably somewhere in between. One study estimates that about 40 per cent of women genuinely suffer premenstrual symptoms.

What *is* unforgivable, at a time when PMT is being seriously discussed at last, are those women who exploit other people's tolerance and blame any passing bitchiness, bloody-mindedness and their own inefficiency on the time of the month. Too many thoughtless excuses and all women will be dumped back into the feeble female stereotype. Anyway, men have moods too – they just haven't a convenient peg to hang them on.

What causes PMT? There's a change in the balance of the female hormones, oestrogen and progesterone, which are at their lowest ebb before a period starts. These are controlled by the same areas of the brain that are affected by factors such as stress, worry, poor nutrition and too much strenuous exercise – one reason women's periods can be so susceptible to life changes. Other culprits include a rise in another hormone, prolactin, and a deficiency of essential fatty acids (EFAs).

Self-help

★ Low progesterone makes the body susceptible to the effects of low blood sugar, which makes tiredness worse. To maintain blood sugar, don't raid the kitchen sugar bowl. True, you'll increase your blood sugar, but too fast – and then it will drop too far and too quickly, like a roller coaster. Eat **small starchy snacks** every three hours instead – wholemeal bread, oatmeal biscuits, crispbread, jacket potato, porridge.

★ Cut down on salt to reduce water retention and on animal fat. Reduce your cups of tea and coffee and other caffeine drinks. Eat plenty of fresh fruit and veg.

★ Consider supplementing your diet with **evening primrose oil.** This (and borage and blackcurrant oil) is stuffed with gammalinolenic acid (GLA) which helps make the hormones called prostaglandins that regulate body functions. For some reason it appears to work brilliantly for some women and not for others.

★ Another supplement to try is **vitamin B6**, which works on the parts of the brain that control depression, although, as with evening primrose oil, research findings are both for and against. **Zinc** and **magnesium** can also help with the blues.

★ Aromatherapists recommend a daily bath with the essential oils of **clary sage, geranium** and **lavender** for two weeks before your period is due – but take care you are not pregnant. These herbs are strong relaxants. Oils of Roman camomile, otto rose and melissa and **camomile tea** are also suggested.

★ Homeopathic remedies include **sepia** if you have tender breasts, depression and loss of libido; **natrum mur.** if you have swollen breasts, irritability and fluid retention.

★ **Acupuncture** and **massage** can also be helpful.

References

Marie Stopes Well Woman Centre,
   PMT Clinic,
   Marie Stopes House,
   108 Whitfield Street,
   London W1P 6BE
   (tel. 071-388 0662)

National Association for Premenstrual Syndrome (NAPS),
   PO Box 72,
   Sevenoaks,
   Kent TN13 1XQ

PMS Help,
   PO Box 160,
   St Albans,
   Herts AL1 4LE

The Premenstrual Society (Premsoc),
  PO Box 429,
  Addlestone,
  Surrey KT15 1DZ

The Women's Nutritional Advisory Service,
  PO Box 268,
  Lewes,
  East Sussex BN7 2QN
  (tel. 0273 487366)

Am I a Monster, Or Is This PMS? by Louise Roddon   (Headline)
Banish PMT and Painful Periods by Elizabeth Martyn (Meadowdale)
Beat PMT Through Diet by Maryon Stewart (Vermilion)
Menstrual and Pre-menstrual Tension by Jan de Vries (Mainstream)

10. Thyroid disorders

Debilitating fatigue and weakness are one of the key signals of an underactive thyroid gland (hypothyroidism). So are – hypochondriacs get ready – constipation, headache, depression, mental confusion, aching muscles, weight gain, unsteadiness when walking, chest pains, shortness of breath, swelling ankles, heavy periods (and hence anaemia), blocked nose, feeling cold, a slurred voice, puffy eyes, thin hair and dry skin, a sore throat and tender and swollen glands, a slow pulse and raised blood pressure. Have I left anything out? Yes – six out of seven sufferers are women.

The thyroid produces an iodine-rich hormone whose main ingredient is thyroxin. It is responsible for the body's metabolism and therefore mental and physical growth and development, and is controlled in turn by the pituitary gland which secretes the thyroid stimulating hormone.

Once diagnosed – a blood test usually confirms that fairly definitive list of symptoms – treatment is prompt and effective: thyroxin (or T4) tablets for the rest of your life.

Self-help
Kelp and iodine-rich food such as sea fish, vegetables, milk
and meat can be beneficial. So may vitamins C, B3 and B5,
and minerals manganese, calcium and zinc, which are important for the functioning of the thyroid and pituitary gland.
Homeopathy and reflexology are worth looking into.

11. Drugs
Don't forget that the side effects of many drugs prescribed
include fatigue – and some of them for conditions in which
fatigue is a symptom! These pharmaceuticals include: anticon-
vulsants, antidepressants, tranquillisers and hypnotics (especially benzodiazepines, such as Valium and Mogadon),
antihistamines (such as hayfever preparations and cold remedies), beta blockers, drugs for diabetes and high blood pressure, diuretics, muscle relaxants, and over-the-counter
preparations containing codeine (such as painkillers and cough
mixtures).

Don't hurl them down the loo in despair though. They could
be keeping you alive. Ask your doctor if there's an alternative
that has less tiring side effects.

The contraceptive pill – especially the progestogen-only pill
(POP or mini-pill) – may cause fatigue, depression and a lack of
interest in sex in some women.

Of course, in talking about drugs don't forget the social kind
that most of us throw down our throats every day – alcohol and
caffeine-rich tea, chocolate, cola drinks and coffee. A cup of
coffee mid-morning enhances concentration (as a mildly
addicted coffee drinker I would say that of course, but recent
research agrees). Too much coffee however (and for some
people three cups a day is an overdose) has been known to
produce anxiety, nervous disorders and fatigue.

References

The Wellness Encyclopaedia, The University of California,
Berkeley (Houghton Mifflin)

The New Our Bodies, Ourselves, Boston Women's Health Book
  Collective (Penguin)
Family Doctor Home Adviser, the British Medical Association
  (Dorling Kindersley)
The New Body Talk by Michael van Straten (Headline)

CHAPTER 3

The alternative route

YOUR LIFESTYLE

If there is no physical reason discovered for your tiredness, and you're blessed in your GP, he or she will ask you about your lifestyle. Are you working too hard? Do you have financial problems? Are the children being difficult? Because fatigue, when there is no medical explanation, is often – invariably – the result of something askew in our lives. The balanced interaction between rest and work and play and loving and caring that we need for optimum health has somehow come unstuck.

Our society being what it is – materialist, competitive, status-conscious, technology-crazy – overwork is often to blame. But equally, tiredness can be due to not enough work, to boredom. Or to an excess of caring – mothers who can't let grown up children fly the nest, who need to find an identity of their own. Or it can be, quite pragmatically, as with students, the result of not enough sleep.

It's a sad fact that few GPs have a spare hour or so to talk, because often that's all that is needed to help somebody sort out where their priorities have gone awry. Resist, if you can, prescriptions for tranquillisers or sleeping pills, other than the short term (unless you are referred to a psychiatrist for depression; see Chapter 13). They only sweep the real sources of your fatigue under the carpet; sooner or later it will crawl out again and look just as horrible.

If you're lucky, your doctor may refer you to a psychotherapist or a counsellor. And if you're *exceptionally* fortunate, and your doctor acknowledges that well-being involves not just the state of the body, but the mind and the emotions and the spirit, she may suggest a complementary therapist. But if this is the route you want, in reality you usually have to explore it yourself.

What can complementary medicine offer?
Most of us hate handing over control of our well-being to someone else. It's *our* body, after all. We feed it and groom it, and we'd like to take some responsibility for it, thank you. Fortunately, there's often quite a lot you can do to back up any prescribed drugs or medical care.

'Self-help', 'complementary' and 'holistic' are buzz words that people throw into a kind of alternative health pot, along with other vague ideas like eating more carrots and wholemeal bread and even 'new age' and 'crystals'. Some of it is nonsense, some of it is basic common sense, and quite a bit of it actually works, even if nobody can quite explain why. Yet.

People talk about 'holistic' food, 'holistic' cosmetics, even 'holistic' holidays without really thinking about the meaning, but the dictionary defines it as 'relating to organic and functional relations between parts and a whole'. Hmmm. Holistic health therefore means that the well-being of the whole – in this case, you or me – depends on the fitness of each of our component parts.

Mind, body, and spirit are so threaded together that it is almost impossible to disentangle them, as modern science is discovering. When one strand is sick, it affects the others; to enhance one can energise the rest. So if we're going to be as healthy and as full of vitality as we can, it's not simply a question of watching our blood pressure, exercising twice a week and getting eight (or seven, or whatever) hours' sleep a night. It's keeping our brain active, allowing our emotions natural expression and seeking to find the best in ourselves and others.

Complementary medicine has always understood the importance of treating the whole patient, not just the bit that's sick. True healing comes from within, when the body's own battalions are summoned into action. Not only must our immune systems be ready to fight disease, but all our vital energies, whether of the flesh or the spirit, flow unimpeded.

The vast majority of therapies also work well with orthodox medicine; it's rarely a case of either/or, although it's a good idea to let your doctor know of any treatment you are receiving from a complementary therapist.

Some GPs can get rather sniffy about what they call 'quackery', but there has been an astonishing increase in the number of doctors referring patients to practitioners in the more 'acceptable' (i.e., least at odds with Western science) therapies, such as homeopathy, acupuncture and traditional Chinese medicine, especially now that they are able to make payments for them out of their practice budgets. Your GP may even be one of those who share their practice with several complementary therapists.

Otherwise you're on your own. Some treatments, such as Bach Flower Remedies, you can follow for yourself, but for others you'll need to find a qualified practitioner. Be prepared to pay *at least* £20 for a treatment, though costs vary according to the therapy, length of session and which area you live in. In London, an hour's aromatherapy massage could be £25, a consultation with a homeopathic doctor £50.

The daunting question is how to find the correct practitioner. Which is the best therapy for you? And what, exactly, are meant by qualifications? This question exercises the entire complementary medical world, let alone some poor tired individual who doesn't know an essential oil from a decoction.

Can you be sure your alternative therapist is safe?

You should be relatively confident if your GP refers you to a therapist, but otherwise, how can you be sure that the person you're entrusting with your body and mind really knows what they're doing? Do those initials after their name really mean anything? It depends. 'There's nothing to stop anybody going on a weekend course and then putting up a sign for business as a therapist,' snaps one resentful counsellor, with years of

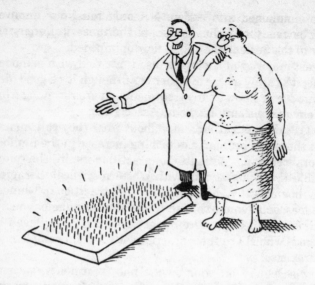

training and experience unrecognised by the general public.

With the exception of osteopathy, which Parliament established as a registered medical profession last year, there are no Government requirements for training in complementary medicine.

Conscious of the European Commission's more rigorous attitude and the very real health risk from irresponsible cowboys (one leading practitioner dramatically describes the situation as a 'health disaster just waiting to happen'), reputable complementary therapies are desperately trying to form voluntary registering bodies to set training and practice standards. But how do you devise regulations that will satisfy staid and well-behaved disciplines like homeopathy, and exotic fringe therapies such as dowsing and crystal healing?

If in any doubt, ask the therapist what her letters stand for and check them out with the following organisations: the Council for Complementary and Alternative Medicine represents the more mainstream therapies – acupuncture, homeopathy, medical herbalism and traditional Chinese medicine. The

British Complementary Medicine Association lists approved training bodies for a wide range of therapies, from aromatherapy to colour healing.

References

British Complementary Medicine Association,
 St Charles Hospital,
 Exmoor Street,
 London W10 6DZ
 (tel. 081-964 1205)

Council for Complementary and Alternative Medicine,
 179 Gloucester Place,
 London NW1 6DX
 (tel. 071-724 9103)

What do complementary therapies involve? And how can they help those of us who feel tired all the time? In the last chapter, I suggested possible complementary treatments for the various complaints. Many therapies offer remedies for fatigue – though most will seek to uncover *why* you are so exhausted. Here is a *brief* rundown on the better known ones:

ACUPUNCTURE

You've probably seen rather unnerving photographs of people undergoing acupuncture, with clusters of long thin needles projecting from various parts of their body. (It doesn't hurt, they all insist reassuringly.) According to this ancient Chinese therapy, the body's energy or vital force (known as Qi, pronounced 'chi') circulates through a series of invisible channels, or meridians, which are linked to our internal organs. When we are sick, Qi is blocked, and the needles (which in most cases only penetrate the skin by a few millimetres – no blood!) are said to unblock, increase or decrease the flow of Qi.

43

Good health is also maintained by keeping two opposing but complementary forces, yin (female) and yang (male) in balance. Yin is passive, tranquil, dark, moist, cold, and swelling. Too much of it causes aches, pains, discharges, fluid retention and tiredness. Yang, on the other hand, is aggressive: light, heat, dryness, contraction. An excess can bring on headaches and high blood pressure.

Because acupuncturists believe that tiredness is due to a malfunction of the internal organs, they would apply needles to points on the meridians regulating these. Moxibustion – in which *Qi* is boosted by burning a cone of plant wool on the end of the needle – might be suggested.

The Council for Acupuncture has a register of qualified acupuncturists (as anyone can legally use the title 'acupuncturist', it's important to find someone who knows what they're doing). Look for qualifications MBAcA, FBAcA, LicAc, BAc, DrAc.

Reference

The Council for Acupuncture,
 179 Gloucester Place,
 London NW1 6DX
 (tel. 071-724 5756)

AROMATHERAPY

One of the most popular of complementary therapies, and no wonder – what could be more delicious than a soothing massage with heavenly smelling oils? Certain plant extracts – the essences or essential oils – are believed to have specific healing properties which are absorbed by the skin. When used in massage they are diluted in vegetable oil or alcohol (never put concentrated oils directly on the skin or swallow them, unless advised by a trained aromatherapist), or add a few drops to your bath before a good soak. The scent is also an important part of the healing – scientists have shown certain smells act directly on the brain (See Chapter 12.)

If you're physically knocked out, aromatherapists suggest inhaling stimulating essential oils, such as black pepper, lemon, lemon grass and rosemary, from a tissue, or adding a few drops to a warm bath. Try clary sage, rosemary and savory for mental fatigue.

References

To find a qualified practitioner, contact:
International Federation of Aromatherapists,
  Dept. of Continuing Education,
  The Royal Masonic Hospital,
  London W6 0TN
  (tel. 081-846 8066)

Aromatherapy Organisations Council,
  3 Latymer Close,
  Braybrooke,
  Market Harborough,
  Leics. LE16 8LN

The Aromatherapy Workbook by Shirley Price (Thorsons)

BACH FLOWER REMEDIES

Dr Edward Bach, an eminent physician and homeopath practising in London at the beginning of the century, believed that flowers could affect the state of mind and restore the natural harmony necessary for good health. He identified 38 preparations, which had to be obtained in a very particular way.

At first only the dew on flowers was 'impregnated' with their healing properties; later – dew being difficult to bottle in quantity – he decided that clear spring water on which freshly picked flowers had floated in sunlight would do as well.

Try hornbeam as a remedy for mental fatigue and the Monday morning feeling; olive for exhaustion and feeling drained of energy by intractable problems.

Reference

Dr Edward Bach Centre,
  Mount Vernon,
  Sotwell,
  Wallingford,
  Oxon OX10 0PZ
  (tel. 0491 834678)

CHIROPRACTIC

Back pain, neck pain and headaches that cause fatigue have been successfully treated by chiropractics, who manipulate the body – and especially the spine – to restore normal function to joints and muscles. McTimoney is a gentle form of chiropractic that involves a shorter training course.

References

British Chiropractic Association
  29 Whitley Street,
  Reading RG2 0EG
  (tel. 0734 757557)

Institute of Pure Chiropractic (McTimoney),
  14 Park End Street,
  Oxford OX1 1HH
  (tel. 0865 246687)

HERBALISM

Herbalism – using the natural healing properties of plants – has become increasingly popular as people have grown aware of the environment and ecology, and leery of the side effects of synthetic drugs. What is natural must be good. That doesn't automatically mean harmless, however – comfrey got a bad press recently when a woman who took it without supervision suffered liver damage – and it's important to consult a trained medical herbalist and not buy any old herb over the counter.

Like most complementary therapies, herbalism treats the patient holistically as an individual, not as a disease. A herbalist will take a careful case history to determine what underlying problem could be causing your symptoms, before prescribing herbs to flush out your toxins and restore your body to its normal balance in order to heal itself.

Herbs that can ease fatigue include basil, lemon balm, rosemary and sage. Make a herbal infusion by warming a teapot and putting in one dessertspoon of fresh or dried herb for each cup required. Pour in a cup of boiling water for each cup of tea, and allow to steep for 10–15 minutes.

Send s.a.e. to the Honorary Secretary, National Institute of Medical Herbalists for a list of herbalists.

Reference

National Institute of Medical Herbalists,
  9 Palace Gate,
  Exeter EX1 1JA
  (tel. 0392 426022)

HOMEOPATHY

Homeopathy works on the principle of 'like cures like'. This means that a substance which causes certain symptoms in a healthy person can cure someone who has developed similar symptoms as the result of a disease. (Sounds complicated, but read the sentence again slowly.)

Arsenic, for example, which as any reader of thrillers knows is horribly fatal, is a homeopathic remedy for diarrhoea or vomiting from food poisoning. The remedies are completely safe, because they are diluted thousands of times over until there are only a few molecules, if any, of the original substance left; in fact, homeopaths believe that the weaker the dilution the more potent the remedy. Somehow the substance leaves 'footprints' in the dilution. Of course, this defies any current scientific explanation, so many orthodox doctors dismiss it as nonsense.

Nonetheless hundreds of thousands of people swear by homeopathy, including the British Royal Family, and several scientifically controlled trials have been carried out which indicate that homeopathy really does work, especially in treating hayfever and asthma.

Symptoms such as fatigue are regarded as signs of imbalance within the whole person. The skill of the homeopath lies in matching as many of the patient's symptoms, habits and personality traits to one of two thousand remedies available. For this reason, an initial consultation can take an hour to an hour and a half, during which the homeopath asks detailed questions about what you eat, what time you go to bed, what your likes and dislikes are. Researchers suggest this may be one reason homeopathy is successful. Psychologically, people feel better because the practitioner is taking a genuine interest in them, rather than wondering if the waiting room will be emptied before lunch.

If you can't sleep after a lot of physical activity, try two or three doses of Arnica 30. Phosphorus three times a day for three weeks might restore lost energy after a long period of study or strain (students please note!) For mental or physical depression or lack of nerve power, try two or three doses of Kali carb.

References

The British Homeopathic Association,
27a Devonshire Street,
London W1N 1RJ
(tel. 071-935 2163)
(s.a.e. for list of doctors who are homeopaths)

The Family Guide to Homeopathy by Dr Andrew Lockie
(Hamish Hamilton)

HYPNOTHERAPY

If you've seen a stage hypnotist persuade people to make fools of
themselves, then forget it. The kind of trance a hypnotherapist
will induce is very light – just enough for him or her to communicate suggestions to your unconscious without your conscious mind
interfering. It's very relaxing; you usually lie back in a comfortable chair, and a qualified hypnotherapist would no more take
advantage of your susceptibility than fly. You're invariably aware
of what's happening anyway.

Apart from giving up smoking, drugs and alcohol, hypnotherapy has been successful in treating skin disorders,
migraine, peptic ulcers, irritable bowel syndrome and other
stress fallout complaints. It won't cure tiredness as such, but
it can alleviate the conditions exacerbating your fatigue.

Reference

British Society of Medical and Dental Hypnosis,
17 Keppel View Road,
Kimberworth,
Rotherham,
South Yorkshire S61 2AR
(tel. 0709 554558)

NATUROPATHY

Disease is due to a breakdown in your natural healthy balance,
and treatment is aimed at building up your resources so that
you can bounce back. It was naturopaths who first sang the
praises of high-fibre food, and drew attention to the dangers of
pesticides and food additives. Most advice is about diet – eat

more salads, drink less coffee, et cetera – and sometimes fasting is recommended. Don't ever do this off your own bat; always consult a qualified naturopath.

Naturopaths treat each patient as an individual, taking into account their entire physical, emotional, biochemical and social circumstances. Any advice about feeling tired all the time would therefore vary from one person to another.

References

General Council and Register of Naturopaths
  (tel. 0458 2103377)

British Naturopathic Association,
  Frazer House,
  6 Netherhall Gardens,
  London NW3 5RR
  (tel. 071-435 8728)

OSTEOPATHY

Low back pain, neck pain and tension headaches – a source of fatigue – often respond well to osteopathy. When the body is well-tuned it will purr along like a Rolls Royce, say osteopaths. They massage and manipulate your body with their hands to get bones, joints, muscles and ligaments functioning normally again. Akin to chiropractic, it puts less emphasis on the spine, and relies less on X-rays and conventional diagnostic methods.

References

General Council and Register of Osteopaths,
  56 London Street,
  Reading,
  Berkshire RG1 4SQ

Osteopathic Information Service,
 37 Soho Square,
 London W1V 5DG
 (tel. 071-439 7177)

General References

Reader's Digest Guide to Alternative Medicine
The Handbook of Complementary Medicine by Stephen Fulder
 (Coronet, Hodder & Stoughton)
British Holistic Medical Association *Tapes for Health* (subjects
 include insomnia, pain, visualisation, stress, relaxation)
 179 Gloucester Place,
 London NW1 6DX
 (tel. 071-262 5299)

CHAPTER 4

Is it really ME?

ME

'It's ME,' says the sufferer feebly from her sofa. 'I'm totally exhausted. I can hardly get myself downstairs to make a cup of tea. Life's not worth living.'

We see them, these victims – or read about them, more likely, as it is in the nature of their condition to be prostrate, confined to their palliasses. Pale wraith-like figures who can barely struggle to answer the telephone: for whom the ordinary demands of life, their job, their family, are wearying beyond measure. 'Tired' can't describe it enough. This is FATIGUE in capital letters. Even those of us dragging around with TATT can't rise – or more appropriately, sink – to their spectacular levels of debilitation.

Are they putting it on? Those in rude health must admit to a passing irritation at their complaints. 'I can't come to dinner, I must rest.' 'I won't be at work, my doctor's given me a medical certificate for another month.' What a lurk, we think uncharitably. What he/she needs is a good kick up the . . . well, you know. This is grossly unfair, because their symptoms are very real and utterly devastating, as any sufferer or their family will confirm.

ME became the vogue disease of the eighties. 'Yuppie flu' the media called it, because it tends to strike successful hard-working people in their twenties and thirties, transforming them overnight into limp shadows of their former selves. What starts as a cold or bout of flu refuses to go away. Months, even years, later people are still unable to get about and live normally, and yet doctors can find no sign of a recognisable disease. What the hell is going on?

For a start, the name ME – myalgic encephalomyelitis – is a misnomer. The term means inflammation of the brain and the spinal cord with associated muscular pain, a condition not apparent in most alleged ME sufferers.

In many cases, tests show nothing: no funny cells, no marauding bacteria, no alien viruses, nothing to explain the overwhelming lethargy, mental exhaustion, muscle and chest pains, twitching limbs, itchy rashes, sweating, panic attacks, memory loss, nausea, insomnia, swollen glands, fever, shivering fits, ringing in the ears and all the other myriad symptoms of which sufferers complain.

The medical profession has problems defining this mysterious illness. There's no diagnostic test and it's hard to get an agreement on symptoms, or how many people suffer from it – 100,000 people in the UK is one estimate. Despite being recognised as an illness by the Department of Health and Social Security, which means victims can at least claim benefits, a hard core of doctors still dismisses its existence. 'Malingering', 'all in the mind' or 'clinical depression' they grumble, which drives ME patients into as violent a paroxysm of fury as their lack of energy will allow.

Is it one disease or many?
But getting to grips with the syndrome isn't easy, and it's not helped by the plethora of names that accumulate around it. Are we talking about ME, or Chronic Fatigue Syndrome (CFS), or Epstein-Barr, or Royal Free disease (after an outbreak among staff and patients at the Royal Free Hospital, London, in the 1950s) or Post Viral Fatigue Syndrome (PVFS), or Persistent Virus Disease? Are they different conditions that happen to share fatigue as a symptom – or all the same thing?

A self-perpetuating industry has mushroomed: books are written, patients' associations and support groups proliferate; conferences, seminars, research organisations, and remedy manufacturers all beaver away. Whatever the enigma is (as international experts have agreed to call it Chronic Fatigue Syndrome so will I, though in Britain it's still commonly known as ME – despite a lobby to rename it Persistent Virus Disease) a lot of people now have a vested interest in its existence.

There are some clues. Researchers have found abnormalities in the immune system and especially the muscle cells of some sufferers. Certain viruses are on the suspect list: the eloquently titled Coxsackie B and a swarm of enteroviruses that spawn in the bowels. Epstein-Barr and cytomegalovirus are the herpes viruses responsible for glandular fever, the infectious disease most common among adolescents whose immune defences are not fully developed; victims usually recover in six weeks or so, but may feel tired and depressed for several months afterwards. In the US, they're excited about exotic retroviruses, more elusive and harder to detect than an ordinary old virus. And it seems that a newly discovered herpes virus is more common among chronic fatigue patients. Another possibility could be parasitic infestations in the gut. Two likely candidates are giardia lamblia and blastocystis hominis, charmers that worm their way in via tap water or human contact. Only expensive laboratory tests can detect them. Orthodox medicine uses powerful drugs to flush them out but medical herbalists report success with hefty doses of natural herbs. The bottom line, however, as most experts agree, is that *no* single factor leads to CFS in all patients.

All in the mind?

On the other hand, the fact that antidepressants can make a difference for many sufferers – one doctor says 80 per cent of her patients improve on taking them – points to a psychological factor. Cases of what 19th-century doctors called neurasthenia (nervous exhaustion with no definite disease) bear a creepy resemblance to some modern examples.

Victorian doctors called them 'bed cases' or 'sofa cases'. It was very fashionable for upper middle-class ladies to complain of fatigue and muscle weakness and take to their beds. 'Weak, pallid, flabby . . . poor eaters; digesting ill, incapable of exercise . . . They lie in bed, or on sofas, hopeless and helpless, and exhibit every conceivable variety of hysteria,' wrote an unsympathetic society physician in 1881.

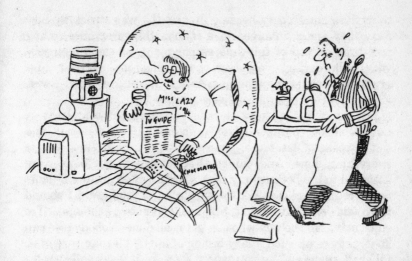

A 36-year-old German woman, in bed for eleven years because of fatigue and muscle weakness, was admitted to a private sanatorium in Berlin in 1867. She disliked light, the doctor noted, and she spoke slowly and tonelessly, without energy. He prescribed a routine of hot baths and lots of psychological encouragement, and (no prizes for guessing) before long she rose from her bed and walked.

CFS may not have a straightforward physical cause, some experts now suspect. It's a 'lifestyle' disease, another example of the interconnectedness of mind and body. The symptoms, the exhaustion, the aches and pains, are real enough, but at an unconscious level the mind allows – or even manipulates – the body to be sick. Immune system defences are dropped and invading viruses slip through. The question is why does this happen.

OVERLOAD ESCAPE?

Norma Ware, an anthropologist at Harvard Medical School, recently interviewed Chronic Fatigue Syndrome patients about their lives before they became ill, and she was struck by how *busy* they were: 'involved in a million things at once, piling part-time on top of full-time employment, or combining jobs with childrearing, volunteer work, vigorous exercise programmes, caring for ageing parents and active social lives'. Eighty per cent of sufferers were women.

But it's by no means an exclusively feminine complaint. A man reported: 'I was working probably 60 hours a week and some weeks a lot more. There wasn't enough time to get everything done. And things that needed to get done were assigned to me because my boss knew I would get them done. So he really loaded me down with a lot of stuff. And I should have said "no", but I didn't, because, you know, I thought, "I'm superman. I'm the guy who can get it all done. Nobody else can do it; they're all such a lazy bunch of idiots. I'll take care of it. I'll show them all." In retrospect, I mean, it was really pretty dumb.'

More intriguingly, Dr Ware sees Chronic Fatigue Syndrome as a mass reaction to pressures in modern Western society. People expect – and are expected – to do too much. We're *proud* of being over-extended, pulled in fifty different directions, always in a rush. Look how in demand we are. How cleverly we cope. How well we squeeze it all in. Holidays are for wimps, only the uncommitted leave the office at five.

Sometimes the only escape from this rat race is to get sick. Physically sick. Dr Ware found that, for nearly half of her interviewees, chronic fatigue syndrome was a catalyst that enabled them to adopt a radical new lifestyle. It gave them permission to stop working 60 or 80 hours a week. They eventually learnt to relax, to allow themselves some leisure, to care about other people, to stop 'doing' and think about 'being'. Ultimately they regained control of their life, and this time ran things the way *they* wanted.

It's a pretty drastic way out. All that pain and misery, all that disability and despair. And yet so many patients described the experience as ultimately 'good' for them.

'I don't want to say it was a blessing in disguise, because that sounds horrible – "I'm glad to get sick," ' one told Dr Ware. 'But in some ways I'm sort of glad it got me out of all these problems and really turned me around to say, "Hey, you're not happy and you're going to have to do something to change." I hate to say the word "grateful", but in some ways, I am.'

Reference

Chronic Fatigue Syndrome, Ciba Foundation Symposium 173, (John Wiley & Sons)

'I'm not nuts'
Nevertheless, many CFS sufferers loathe *any* kind of psychological tag. When patients at a London hospital were referred to a psychiatrist they went up the wall. How dare the doctors imply their illness was imaginary: 'I'm not nuts, I'm *really* ill,' they insisted.

There's still a stigma attached to anything that could seem a mental weakness and – it must be whispered – medical insurance and disability benefits are higher for physical than psychological disorders. 'Psychosomatic' somehow implies it's all your fault; but a virus now, who can help that?

Personality may have a hand in the situation too, which won't please some patients. Not when they learn that those considered most likely to collapse with CFS are introverted, neurotic, emotionally vulnerable and depressive.

Nor will you get better if you have the wrong attitude, is the brisk opinion of many psychiatrists. Rest is the best way to alleviate the symptoms of CFS, and it's sensible not to overtax yourself, but *some* exercise, however mild, is beneficial. Patients are sometimes told to stay in bed, which can be physically disastrous.

'You lose 10 per cent of muscle power after a week's bedrest,' says a London psychiatrist specialising in CFS. 'When healthy young men spend three weeks in bed, their fitness falls by a third. If you're in bed for months, you'll be as weak as a kitten. Of course you'll feel awful and have aches and pains.

'If you're a passive victim and you think you can't do anything, or you're frightened of a relapse, you'll stay in bed, get depressed and physically unfit. You'll have trouble sleeping and get iller and iller, and end up in a wheelchair.' Horrendous thought. Is this how someone feeling a bit low after glandular fever can end up depressed and bedridden eight months later, clinging to the CFS or ME label for grim death?

Apparently. But, he adds, if patients can admit, ' "Yes, I have a stressful life at the moment, and yes, I have a virus, but I need to change the direction of my life; I need to spend time with my partner," or "I wouldn't go back to that job even if I was well," then I know they'll get better.'

ARE THESE YOUR SYMPTOMS?

The US Federal Center for Disease Control and Prevention's definition of CFS (aka ME and PVFS) has been accepted by most international experts.

If you have the energy to work out their checklist, chances are you don't have it.

Part A: Prolonged (lasting six months or more) or recurring, severely debilitating fatigue that cuts one's activity level to 50 per cent or less of what it was previously

AND

Part B: Other conditions that may produce similar symptoms must be excluded. These include: malignancy; autoimmune disease; localised infections; chronic or subacute bacterial disease, fungal disease and parasitic disease; disease related to HIV infection; chronic psychiatric

disease, either newly diagnosed or by history; chronic
inflammatory disease; neuromuscular disease; endocrine
disease; drug dependency or abuse; side effects of a chronic
medication or other toxic agent; or other known or defined
chronic pulmonary, cardiac, gastrointestinal, liver, kidney
or blood disease

AND

Part C: Eight of the following 11 symptoms:

1.   Low-grade fever
2.   Sore throat
3.   Painful lymph nodes in the neck or underarms
4.   Muscle weakness
5.   Muscle pain
6.   Prolonged fatigue after exercise
7.   Headaches
8.   Migratory joint pain without swelling or redness
9.   One or more of: light sensitivity, forgetfulness, irrita-
     bility, confusion, difficulty thinking or concentrating,
     depression
10. Sleep disturbances
11. Abrupt onset of symptoms

OR

If you currently have at least 6 of the above 11 symptoms
and can prove you have had at least 2 of the 3 below:

1.   Low-grade fever
2.   Inflamed throat
3.   Palpable or tender lymph nodes in neck or armpits

'MIRACULOUSLY I BEGAN TO FEEL BETTER'

'The tiredness started with a virus infection three years ago, when I also had a severe sore throat and pains in my hip joints,' says Elaine, a children's book illustrator. 'Any exertion, particularly walking or climbing stairs and hills exhausted me. Shopping in the supermarket wiped me out so much I had to go to bed, and that would be it for the day.

'I'd wake up tired and force myself out of bed. Halfway through the morning I'd be so shattered I couldn't go on. I'd literally have to go to bed and sleep for an hour, and then maybe have another hour's sleep in the afternoon. Although I was in bed by 9.30p.m. I never seemed to have enough sleep.

'Because I worked from home I could just manage – with buckets of coffee – to carry on. Then I allowed myself to think it was ME. I read up about that, and about candida albicans, and put myself on a diet. No more tea or coffee, dairy products or wheat.

'My GP referred me to a London teaching hospital, where I saw a nice registrar who said (a) my virus was a precipitating factor; (b) I was stressed; and (c) my endocrine system wasn't performing properly. He did some tests but nothing looked even remotely suspicious.

'So then I saw a rheumatologist and an allergy specialist, but still no answer. It was very dispiriting – I carted myself around one outpatients department after another, and all the advice was bitty and never seemed to look at the whole picture.

'It was true I was stressed. I worried about money. Would I get another work assignment? Would my dilapidated house fall down? I had a dear friend who was seriously sick and I hadn't had a proper holiday for years. I just hadn't given myself enough space. I was also menopausal, although I don't know how much this was a factor – none of the doctors seemed to consider it so. My GP suggested HRT, but I didn't feel that was the answer.

'After two years of feeling rough and with no solution in sight, I saw an ME specialist. He said, "You're the type: a perfectionist with a lot of stress from work, inclined to get depressed and introverted. You're working at home and you need to get out and about. You're not sufficiently relaxed to let life take its course. You always want to be in control and that becomes tiring."

'He was right. Lately I've tried to relax, do things like painting and drawing. Yoga has been tremendously helpful. In the meantime I consulted various complementary therapists. An osteopath gave me a lot of time and attention but it got nowhere, and a naturopath was very keen on diet, which was quite good because he could monitor me, but still nothing wonderful.

'I went to an ME group but I felt oh no, this isn't for me. They talked about their different symptoms and the latest viral research, and I didn't want to be labelled as having ME. It might have started with a virus but I've always suspected it was the mind working through the body. That doesn't make it any easier to deal with though – you still feel tired.

'Then a friend suggested I see an acupuncturist. It was shattering to begin with. For the first four sessions everything got worse and I was tempted to give up, and then, miraculously, I began to feel better.

'She's very good at seeing me as a whole person, and she has sorted out my digestion – she said I had irritable bowel syndrome, which is common in post viral fatigue. She prescribed traditional Chinese herbal medicine too – the herbs look beautiful in their package but you boil them up and they taste disgusting. However, it all seems to work – my energy levels are up for the first time in years.

'But I have to pace myself and not overdo it. I've discovered there are different sorts of tiredness. There's a tiredness due to physical exertion, and another due to mental overwork, and I find it harder to bounce back from the latter. I may still need a couple of days in bed if I overdo things mentally.'

IS IT REALLY CFS?

'I've been feeling tired, I must have CFS,' people say, delighted to have found a trendy explanation for their malaise. With such a grab bag of symptoms, so little in the way of diagnostic tests, and so much hype surrounding chronic fatigue syndrome, there's a real danger of misdiagnosis.

I don't want to frighten you, but— 'Anyone who works in this area has heard examples of patients who initially diagnosed themselves or were diagnosed by a doctor who didn't make an adequate medical evaluation,' says a leading Chronic Fatigue Syndrome specialist. 'Later it turned out they really had leukaemia or ovarian cancer or a psychiatric disorder.'

'When you hear hoofbeats, think horses, not zebras,' is an old medical school saying. Chronic Fatigue Syndrome, says Dr Mark Rapaport of the University of California, is definitely a 'zebra', that should only be diagnosed after more common problems have been ruled out, such as hypothyroidism, vitamin or iron deficiency anaemia, cancer, and psychological disorders, especially depression.

Marilyn, a social worker, went to her GP complaining of 'the most appalling fatigue. The effort of picking up the children from school would send me to bed. If we were going out in the evening, I'd spend the day lying down to save my energy.

' "Post viral fatigue," the doctor said, but I hadn't had a virus. It started after an attack of sunstroke on holiday in Menorca. Then I saw a psychologist who said "depression".

' "I'm not depressed," I said. There's a total difference between depression when you don't want to do *anything*, and the kind of fatigue I had. I *wanted* to get up and go out, do things with the family, but I physically *couldn't*.

'Finally I saw a CFS expert at the School of Hygiene and Tropical Medicine, and he said "I think it's your pituitary; go and see an endocrinologist."

'Well, he was right. The pituitary gland is the master gland of the body, what they call the "conductor of the endocrine orchestra," and mine had stopped producing enough adrenocorticotrophic hormone, known as ACTH, which stimulates the adrenal glands to secrete adrenalin. No wonder I was physically knackered all the time. Now I take steroids, which is a bore, and I'm okay, but I have to be careful not to overdo things.'

References

ME Action,
  PO Box 1302,
  Wells,
  Somerset BA5 2WE
  (tel. 0749 670799)

ME Association,
  Stanhope House,
  High Street,
  Stanford-le-Hope,
  Essex SS17 0HA
  (tel. 0375 642466 fax. 0375 360256)

Living With ME by Dr Charles Shepherd (Heinemann Cedar)

CHAPTER 5

Is your environment getting you down?

SICK BUILDING SYNDROME

I used to work in a building renowned for being unhealthy. At least, we – the employees – claimed it was so ('This building is sick,' we said loudly) but as we worked for a cluster of women's magazines we tended to be rather more clued up on information about the Sick Building Syndrome than most.

None of this cut much ice with the management. It is still an awful place to spend a working day. The air is stuffy and has an over-breathed quality, and viral infections steadily work their way through one staff member after another. People congregate in the loo to compare symptom progress: 'I had the sore throat last week, I'm now on the fever and coughing.' By the end of the day, I would feel like Alice in Wonderland's dormouse, looking for its teapot – tired and sleepy and unable to concentrate.

Escape by opening the windows was impossible. These were bolted shut, so we stared longingly at blue sky and sunshine through tinted glass. One gloriously hot summer's day the air conditioning broke down. People gasped and complained to the managing director's office, and lo, men in overalls came round and unbolted the windows.

We rushed to sample the air that blew across the desks. And what did we find? It was hot and heavy with dust and the fumes of tar and junk food and petrol; the wind blew our papers out of order, and the roar of car engines and the voices of the crowds distracted us. Slowly, slowly, the windows inched shut, until we were safely, hermetically, sealed inside again.

Which was worse? The toxins of re-cycled air, photocopier fumes, and furnishing chemicals? Or the lead and carbon monoxide of the city traffic? Hard to tell – but I appreciated the toll of working in a modern urban environment when I returned to freelance writing at home. For the first time in years I had the energy to read and write after supper in the evening, instead of staring numbly at the television.

Now, if I have occasion to spend a day in that magazine office, I notice how my attention span shortens, fatigue sets in and my head aches. The final killer of course, the whammy to do one in completely, is the journey home on the London Underground at peak hour. There's unhealthy for you: noise, fumes, pollution, crowding, all in a twice-daily megadose.

THE FATIGUE VILLAINS

Environmental pollution is a major cause of fatigue – and doubtless other unspeakable complaints. Some offices should be labelled 'dangerous for your health'. But where do all the toxins come from? And what are the stresses and strains in your workplace that can wring you out?

★ **Air conditioning systems** filter and recirculate air, and maintain a comfortable 24°–27°C, optimum temperature for efficiency. Well, that's the theory. The trouble is that once impurities – carbon monoxide and other toxic gases, air ions, foul odours, viruses and bacteria – get into this mix, they also go round and round. Sore eyes, mysterious allergies, dry skin, headaches and endless respiratory infections (most serious being Legionnaires' Disease) are all part of the fallout.

Central heating dries moisture from the air, which is very draining on the brain and body. You can counteract this with a **humidifier**, or – not quite as efficient, but cheap and simple – a saucer or bowl of water on the radiator.

★ **Air ions** are positively and negatively charged particles

65

which can affect brain hormones that make you sleepy and sluggish. Fresh air is rich in negative ions, especially by the sea and in the mountains, which help keep you calm and clear-headed.

Positive ions abound in cities, in heavy traffic and 'sick' offices. An excess can make you irritable and depressed.

Ionisers balance the ion levels, replacing positive with negative ions. They're compact, reasonably priced, easily available from high street shops, and on your desk, in your car, or beside your bed at night can make a world of difference to your mood and energy levels.

★ **Formaldehyde** is the demon in the piece. A colourless gas with a pungent odour, it's used to make insulating foam and the glue in particle board, plywood and other wood products used in construction. Some cosmetics, upholstery, permanent press fabrics, carpets and pesticides contain it. You'll also find it in tobacco smoke and the exhaust from certain appliances. When dosed with *huge* amounts, laboratory animals develop cancer. In infinitely smaller doses, humans report burning eyes, itching, shortness of breath, tightness in the chest, coughing, headaches, nausea and asthma attacks.

★ Did it occur to you that the humble **photocopier** in the corner could be leaking **ozone**, a gas given off by high-voltage machines? In reasonable amounts this is okay, but too much can irritate the respiratory system and cause sore throats and laboured breathing.

★ Photocopier toners and drums also contain potentially dangerous chemicals. The intense light can cause eyestrain if not covered, and the noise is a pain if the machine is too close to your workspace.

★ **Noise** is a form of pollution that people can find very wearisome. Machines whine, telephones jangle, voices clatter, air conditioning hums. At the right level, music can help cut out the din and aid concentration – provided you have some control over it and you're not distracted by someone's else blaring CD player or radio. Tuning into your own personal stereo is one way of drowning out the racket and carving out mental space for yourself.

★ **VDUs** are blamed for just about everything: fatigue, eye-strain, blurred vision, sore necks and backs, insomnia, head-aches, nausea, irritability, tension and RSI (repetitive strain injury) in the hands, wrists and forearms. And they're sus-pected of emitting radiation (no worse than that of a fluores-cent light) and causing miscarriages and birth defects (the evidence is uncertain, but using them less than 20 hours a week seems safe).

It's true they're guilty of causing mental and physical fatigue, but the way you sit and how you position your keyboard and screen can do a lot to prevent it.

Fortunately employers are now aware of this and ready to invest money in office furniture. A European Commission Directive on workplace health and safety prodded some into action. Others learnt the hard way: productivity and profits tumbled as staff called in sick with back pain, migraines and stress-related illnesses, and unions complained about workers' RSI.

Job satisfaction appears to protect against these effects – another instance of the mind's influence on the body. People happy in their jobs report fewer VDU-related symptoms.

FIT YOUR WORKSTATION TO YOUR BODY

Move your chair, screen, keyboard and other material so the most important task is directly in front.

Keyboard:

★ Hold wrists straight, elbows at approximately 90 degrees.
★ Adjust seat and keyboard positions to be comfortable.
★ Don't hammer the keyboard.
★ Don't overstretch fingers – move your whole hand.
★ Don't rest wrists on the keyboard or desk while typing.

Screen:
The top of the screen should be at or just below eye level.

★ Keep the VDU at a comfortable distance.
★ Adjust contrast and brightness to avoid eye fatigue.
★ To reduce reflections on the VDU:
    tilt screen
    use an anti-glare filter
    wear dark clothing.
★ Avoid an unshielded window either in front or behind you.
★ Check that overhead lighting does not reflect on the screen.
★ Keep the screen clean.
★ Arrange an eye test if you continue to suffer fatigue, headaches and eyestrain. The flicker of fluorescent lights can exacerbate the flicker of the screen, and special spectacles are available.

Take a break: No matter how well your workstation is designed, you'll be tired and uncomfortable if you work non-stop for long periods. Stop work, get up and walk around every hour or so, and stand up and stretch every 20 minutes.

ARE YOU SITTING COMFORTABLY?

Without doubt, the most important piece of office furniture for your health and energy is your **chair**. The average office worker spends anything from 25 to 40 hours a week sitting down – not including the time crouched behind the wheel of the car or slumped in front of the telly. This may *sound* restful, but not if your muscles are constantly strained by bad posture. Each day 50,000 people take the day off work because their back hurts – and yet every time we sit down we probably make the problem worse.

Our chairs are the wrong height and the wrong angle, so we hunch over our work, shoulders tensed, the spine pinched, stomach squashed so we can't breathe properly and the blood circulation to our legs is blocked. Awful.

'I thought I would have to give up work altogether,' says George, who swapped his office job for freelance brochure writing at home. 'I was sitting in this rigid four-square chair hour after hour and in despair over tiredness, muscle stiffness, headaches and an almost constant pain in my lower back. It cost a fortune but I splurged on one of those Swedish ergonomic chairs that are designed to support your back, and it's been worth every penny.

'The latest thing is "active" seating. The chair "floats", so it follows your body movements even when you're seated. It swivels and tips forward 8 degrees when I operate the VDU and lounges back 15 degrees on a hydraulic gas cylinder when I want to put my feet up on the desk. Wow. I haven't had a back twinge since – in fact, I don't even *think* about my back, and tiredness just isn't a problem any more.'

The perfect chair

1. If possible, try out any new chair for one day, and preferably two.
2. The seat height should be adjustable so that you can put both feet flat on the ground (if not, use a footrest) and a keyboard at, or just below, elbow height.
3. The seat should have a curved 'waterfall' edge and be deep enough to support the full length of the thighs, but not so deep that there is pressure behind the knees when leaning back.
4. The chair should be wide enough to let you change position comfortably.
5. A forward tilt is more comfortable for VDU users and desk work. (Ideally, your worktop should slope upwards, just like the old Victorian school desks.)
6. Make sure the height and tilt of the chair back are adjustable so that it supports the small of your back.

7.   All adjustment knobs and levers should be easily reach-
      able when sitting down.
8.   A five-legged star base is the most stable. Make the chair
      work for you by using castors or gliders to move between
      desks, and swivelling the seat to change direction, rather
      than twisting your trunk.
9.   Padding on the seat and backrest should be firm and deep,
      and the upholstery non-slip and preferably of natural
      fabric so that it's not sweaty.
10.   Move the telephone closer so you don't have to stretch to
      make calls.

Reference

National Back Pain Association,
   31-33 Park Road,
   Teddington,
   Middlesex TW11 0AB
   (tel. 081-977 5474 fax. 081-943 5318)

SPACE CONTROL

Our work performance can also be affected by the way the
office is laid out. Open plan offices, adored by some managers
because they can see what everyone is doing, are proving
deeply unpopular. Humans are territorial animals and we like
to control access to our personal space.

When Vicky's office went open plan, she found the lack of
privacy threatening. 'I felt I was always vulnerable to
interruption by everyone, from the MD to the office junior,
and I couldn't concentrate on my work because every time I
looked up I was distracted. There was too much stimulation,
and I was exhausted.' She managed to build a 'wall' of
bookshelves and potplants that screened her from the worst
of the hurly burly.

GO FOR GREEN

Vicky's potplants were more than just a screen. Plants 'breathe' in carbon dioxide and return oxygen and moisture to the air. When NASA scientists were looking for ways to keep the air in spaceships clean, they discovered the humble spider plant could actually absorb pollutants. In six hours it reduced the amount of formaldehyde in the air by 85 per cent.

The catch (there would be, wouldn't there) is that you'd need as many as seventy spider plants to 'eat' up *all* the carbon monoxide, nitrogen dioxide and formaldehyde floating about in the average home. Still, ten or twelve are better than nothing.

What works terrifically, however, is a solarium full of plants, breathing like mad, through which the ducted air from central heating and air conditioning units is fed and purged. And you thought those fancy atriums full of greenery in new office buildings were just there to look pretty.

Psychologically plants in offices are A Good Thing. In a bid to improve productivity and lift drooping morale, a US company has installed a 4,200 square-foot indoor winter garden where employees can browse and be refreshed by looking at green leaves.

'Workers who are mentally fatigued are less patient and helpful and more easily distracted, and eventually their fatigue becomes stress,' says American psychologist Dr Stephen Kaplan. 'Nature's power in reducing mental exhaustion is awesome, and failure to incorporate it into the workplace will cause a decline in productivity, civility and competence.' Think of that then, as you water your desktop begonia.

THE INCREDIBLE LIGHTNESS

Penny had been about to see a doctor about TATT when her office was redesigned. In a week she cancelled her appointment. Her new desk was beside a window with a view of the street, instead of an airless cubby hole in the middle of the

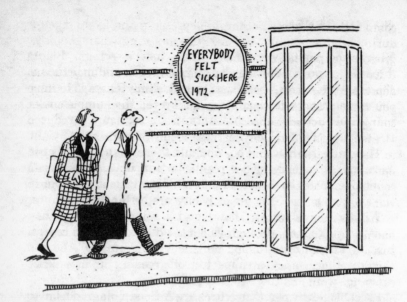

building, blocked from natural light by partitions and illuminated by a fluorescent glare. 'It was almost magic. I felt revitalised, and I no longer come home every night with an aching head.'

In a big office, adjusting the lighting to suit everybody is practically impossible: not too bright, not too dull. VDU users need one kind of light, people who spend a lot of time reading another. Job satisfaction rises with access to natural light, but not *everybody* can squeeze into the top status spot, beside the window. If you're uncomfortable with the light you work by, and can't move your workspace, ask your boss for a desk lamp that throws a gentler light than harsh fluorescent strips above your head.

ARE YOU SAD?

If anything highlights the importance of light, especially sunlight, it's SAD – Seasonal Affective Disorder. SAD people complain of tiredness, lethargy, depression and food bingeing during winter months, and perk up in spring when the days grow longer and lighter.

Every October, Molly would complain of acute fatigue and depression. Her doctor told her she had 'winter blues'. 'Nothing you can do about it,' he said brightly. 'I'll give you another course of antidepressants.'

'I feel as if I'm living in porridge,' Molly complained. 'I want to sleep all the time and it's difficult to get out of bed in the morning. I'm always a bit peckish but I can't be bothered cooking so I top up on biscuits and I've put on a stone. I don't want to go out and meet people, not even the family.'

'I think you've got SAD, Mum,' said Molly's daughter, who had just read a magazine article about it. 'You don't get enough sunlight in the winter so you get tired and depressed.'

It's only in the last five years that the medical profession has eaten its words and acknowledged SAD as a genuine physiological disorder, and not a psychosomatic complaint to shrug off. Sufferers were discovered to have increased levels of the hormone melatonin in their bloodstreams.

Melatonin affects our daily rhythms of sleep and mood. It is secreted by the pineal gland at the base of the brain, and this is stimulated by light entering through the eyes. At night, when we need to be drowsy in order to sleep, melatonin levels rise. At dawn, bright light causes the gland to stop producing the hormone and so we wake up and become active.

People with SAD – probably 1 per cent of the population, and four times as many women as men – are unusually sensitive to reduced sunlight, and can't adapt to the seasonal decrease in winter. Their body clocks slide out of sync with the life they should be leading, and their melatonin levels are only just crawling down at 10 a.m., while everyone else has trained theirs to drop in time for the seven o'clock alarm, even though mornings are dark.

The answer has proved startlingly simple. Light. Or phototherapy, as it's known. The missing daylight is replaced by the necessary amount of bright light. Sitting beside a lightbox that beats out daylight intensity of 2,500 lux for a couple of hours a day is enough to con the pineal gland, and will cure SAD in 86 per cent of patients.

(This is ultraviolet filtered light, by the way, so don't kid yourself you can achieve the same effect by lying on a sunbed. You'll need goggles to avoid eye damage, and these prevent any light reaching the pineal gland – the whole point of the exercise.)

For people in a hurry – who have to get children to school and themselves into the office and haven't the time to twiddle their thumbs in front of a battery of fluorescent tubes – a supersonic version, 10,000 lux, will do the job in 15 or 30 minutes, and sits neatly on a desk.

Latest state-of-the-art equipment is a light visor that sits on your head like a sun helmet. You can walk about while a band of brilliant light beams over your brow. 'Hello earthlings,' you cry. 'This is Captain Zarg from the Planet Zog.'

In the early days of SAD light therapy, full spectrum light was decreed, but subsequent research has shown that simple white light will do the trick as well – and the tubes are considerably cheaper. Prices for a lightbox start at £100, but for someone like Molly it's been worth it: 'I can't believe the difference. My energy levels are the same as in summer, and I've been able to get a part-time job. I watch TV or read a magazine in front of the lightbox – it's no problem.'

Molly had SAD bad (sorry), but 20 per cent of people endure a milder form known as the Winter Blues. In the months between September and March, they feel tired and dreary. Waking up in the morning is hard, they lack energy and enthusiasm for any new projects, and they snack on comfort food a little too much for the good of their waistline.

What they need is an alarm clock with light attached, known as the Dawn Simulator or Natural Alarm Clock. 'The light begins to come on gradually about half an hour before the alarm goes off,' explains its maker, Steve Hayes of Outside In. 'It's a gentle way to wake up that doesn't make you jump, and because it's a gradual brightness it fools the mind that it's a real dawn.'

Blues beaters
Here are some other tips to help banish winter 'blahs'.

★ Avoid sugary snacks that will boost blood sugar and make fatigue worse as well as adding calories. Go for a carbohydrate diet based on whole grains, cereal and wholewheat pasta.
★ Eat seasonal vegetables, rich in beta carotene, and plenty of fruit.
★ Get out in the fresh air as much as possible, and keep an ioniser in your room.
★ Force yourself to take exercise: it will overcome fatigue *and* take off extra weight.
★ Pedalling on an exercise bike in front of your lightbox is said to double the lift.
★ The SAD Association recommends B vitamins, especially B6, and the amino acid food supplement DLPA (DL-phenylalanine), though beware – some people are allergic to it.
★ Treat yourself to an aromatherapy facial with revitalising oils of grapefruit, rose, tangerine and geranium.

Reference

The SAD Association,
  PO Box 989,
  London SW7 2PZ
  (Please send s.a.e. for further information.)

CHAPTER 6

Stressbusting

UNDER STRESS

So you're *still* tired. You've checked out that you don't have anaemia or a food allergy. It's not ME because you can *physically* turn up for work (even if your head remains tucked up in bed) and it's not *just* the office environment, because Monday morning finds you exhausted despite a weekend away from the air conditioning.

The only alternative now is to turn the spotlight on yourself. Look for what experts call 'psychosocial' causes in the way you live. How do you feel about your job, your family, your home, your friends? Are you working too hard? Do you have any control over how you spend your time?

Feeling tired all the time is a major symptom of being stressed. That's right. S.T.R.E.S.S. In fact, the two go hand in hand. If you are stressed – under pressure, tense, worried – then all your systems are in overload and this takes a toll on your mind and body. Just as clapped-out old motor cars and battered aircraft develop metal fatigue, your brain and body are worn out. And that in itself is another source of anxiety.

Because how will you keep meeting your targets when you can't concentrate and you haven't the energy to catch up by putting in extra hours? You're irritable, and the world you inhabit starts to feel like a Salvador Dali painting: slightly surreal, not quite normal. All your vigour is drained by the sheer effort of coping, keeping up appearances, and underneath you're as limp as Dali's infamous drooping watch. Little bits of you literally snap under the strain: your temper, your reasoning ability, your sense of fairness, even your health. No wonder people under pressure are described as 'flaky'.

We make the mistake of blaming stress for the problem, but it's really about how we deal with the *causes* of stress – what experts call the **stressors**. Stress in itself is part of life. Well-maintained airliners are designed to ride out turbulence with ease, and by the same token so are humans. The truth is that we need a certain amount of stimulation, a gingering of challenge, in order to thrive. Good stress – or *eustress*, as it has been called – is the kickstart that enables us to take pride in our work, to make love, and have fun. It's the satisfaction of winning a game of tennis, or completing a job well, and people who are bored or have empty time on their hands show the same symptoms of being stressed as those with too much to do.

Your stressors, however, will not necessarily be mine. The very thought, for instance, of cooking a cordon bleu dinner for ten throws me into a panic; my friend Julia, for whom the kitchen is a place of creative joy, seizes her saucepans with relish. But if the landscape was relatively calm; if there were no looming deadlines, or family dramas, I might think 'hmmm, this could be interesting, something new' and thumb through my recipe books for ideas. My reservoirs of energy would be sufficiently high to take up the challenge.

Too many stressors, though – and this is the situation in which so many people find themselves – and we're like a castle under siege, attacked on all sides; trying to repel the invaders scrambling up the walls, and at the same time to feed and fuel the soldiers on the defence.

'I got one ghastly cold after another,' says Alison, who found herself promoted into a job that was not really her cup of tea. 'Dreadful feverish infections, sore throats, a streaming nose and coughs that I never used to get.'

She was a creative, imaginative woman, a musician who had gone into teaching, and because she was clever and presented herself well – sagacious, intelligent, attractive – she was edged into increasingly administrative posts, until finally she found herself as head of music at a college of higher education. Lots of meetings, lots of decision-taking and telling people what to do, and not very much real music-making.

'I think I was reasonably efficient,' she says, 'so the department didn't fall apart, but it was always a terrible strain. I realised I was literally playing a role, *acting* the part of a manager. I'd think "a manager should wear this", or "a manager would say that", and it was never *me*.'

She might have scraped along like this until retirement – thousands of people do – but for a conglomeration of problems, part work, part personal, that piled up. Her marriage, never a barrel of laughs, was increasingly uncomfortable as her husband's own job came under threat. Her adored 14-year-old son had taken to staying out late at night and communicating in surly grunts. Her bright ten-year-old daughter was falling behind in class. Her mother, who lived alone, was growing forgetful and frail. At college, a new principal was appointed, a man for whom Alison had little respect and even less liking, and the feeling was mutual.

'He seemed out to get me, and because deep down I was insecure in my position, always having to think about what I was doing and lacking any administrative instincts, I became – quite frankly – paranoid. Whenever I counted on getting away from work a few minutes early, in order to be at the school parents' night for instance, he'd call a late meeting. If I took a decision he'd query it. If I wrote a report he'd nitpick through it and want it done again. And the awful thing was that *he* wasn't very competent; he couldn't delegate and he lacked vision. None of us knew where we were going or had any confidence in him.

'Anyway I'd lost my bearings and I seemed to be in a state of constant turmoil. I fretted about every tiny event. I'd come home from work in a horrible mood, shout at the children as soon as I walked in the door, be bad tempered and nag everybody. Why hadn't they put the garbage out? Fed the dog? Did they have to play rock music so bloody loudly? Why wouldn't Rory sit down and eat with us? If my mother rang I snapped at her.

'As for sex with Jim, I was so exhausted when I crawled into bed I couldn't have made love to Tom Cruise if I'd found him between the sheets. I didn't even have the energy to be affectionate, I was so eaten up with all my problems. And I didn't encourage Jim to talk about *his* situation, because I just couldn't take on board another load of angst.

'I'd wake at 4 a.m. and lie awake worrying, holding interminable conversations in my head, planning what to do, what to say, how to behave. I could never get enough sleep – even at weekends I'd still be awake early. I couldn't even relax by zonking out in front of the telly. If I read a magazine I felt guilty. There was always something else I should be doing, and yet I never had the energy to tackle it properly.

'As for my music – what a joke. I hadn't really played in years. I never practised enough, and that became a chore, just another thing I ought to do. I used to belong to a chamber group and I let that go; "too much work, not enough time" I said and felt awful.

'Even the drive to the college and back became a nightmare; I couldn't stand the traffic jams, I worried about whether the car would break down, would I have an accident? Honestly, things I'd never *thought* about before.'

Round and round Alison went: a terrible self-perpetuating cycle of stress feeding on fatigue. In the end, of course, something had to give. She had a panic attack one day in the office, stricken at her desk, shaking with terror, hyperventilating so that her breath came in short pants and pains stabbed her chest. She felt sick and sweaty and dizzy and the walls spun and the floor heaved up and down. She was physically incapable of driving herself home, so her secretary called a taxi.

In the morning the same thing happened when she tried to get ready for work, so she saw the doctor who told her to take three weeks' sick leave and rest. Which she did – and finally had time to think about what was happening in her life.

RED ALERT

If we could see what happens inside our bodies when under threat, we would appreciate why too much of it is tiring.

The first thing you'll encounter in any discussion of stress is the 'fight or flight' response. When our prehistoric ancestors came face to face with a sabre-tooth tiger – a pretty stressful occasion you will agree – their bodies were programmed to survive. Every muscle and nerve rallied so they could respond to danger by either fighting the threat, or getting the hell out of it.

This is the game plan when primitive man spots a tiger, or when his modern counterpart finds himself, for instance, in the path of a speeding car:

★ Extra reserves of the stress hormones – adrenalin, noradrenalin and cortisol – signal battle stations.
★ The heart works faster. Blood pressure rises to pump blood to those parts of the body where it's needed – away from the gut and skin to the muscles of the trunk and limbs.
★ Muscles tense.
★ The liver releases sugar and fats for fast energy.
★ The rate of breathing increases to provide more oxygen.
★ Blood clots more quickly, ready to seal injuries.
★ Digestion stops to divert power to fighting muscles.
★ Saliva dries up.
★ Arteries constrict so that less blood is lost if wounded.
★ Perspiration increases.

That's a hell of a lot of internal action – and if you ever *have* jumped out of real danger, you'll know how suddenly tired and shaky you can feel after a full alert, and how long it can take to return to normal.

So imagine this incredibly complex alarm response system cranking itself up, not for a life-or-death sabre-tooth or even a speeding car, but over a beastly little man in a grey suit, or a crowded train stuck in an Underground tunnel, and doing this hour after hour, day after day. Not always on full red alert, perhaps, but aroused and ready for action – and never quite recovering from one panic before another starts. All that adrenalin bottled up and nowhere to go. You can't thump the Suit, you can't flee the train. Is it any wonder you feel tired?

You may even think that you've become used to stressful situations, and we do adapt to a certain extent – in the same way that people who live beside airports learn to ignore the noise of aeroplanes roaring overhead. But the stress can go underground, and if your reservoir of coping tactics runs low, then up it pops again. Alison, for example, could ignore the myriad little tigers she met driving to and from work – until her reservoir ran dry and she had no extra reserves to buoy her up.

Sometimes we don't even recognise our exhaustion. Jane McWhirter of All Hallows House, a centre for complementary medicine in the City of London, describes people who thrive on such a high level of artificial hype and are so pumped full of adrenalin that they dare not allow themselves to stop in case they sag and can't wind themselves up again.

At weekends when others are enjoying a lazy lie-in, mowing the lawn, saying 'hello birds, hello bees,' and other restful pursuits, these are fretting and twitching and feeling so 'blah' and depressed they can't wait for Monday to throw themselves back into the hurly burly. So addicted are they to a stress 'high' that takes them out of themselves, that a slower pace which allows a glimpse, even a questioning, of the underpinnings is intolerable.

A friend's husband, a high-powered executive who has been known to fly to New York for a meeting and back again the same day, spends his holidays asleep. It's only when he escapes the buzz of the office and sinks down beside a beach or a pool, he says, that the repressed fatigue overwhelms him and then he can't keep his eyes open.

Another City banker, himself grey with exhaustion, describes heavy boardroom meetings where the wheelers and dealers of international finance arrive red-eyed and shaky-handed. These are men who, when big deals are being struck, have barely slept for three days, who have flown halfway across the world and gone straight into top-line negotiations. Who've even had a meeting on the *plane*, for heaven's sake.

Now, no one is so rich or clever or famous that they don't get tired, and that's when chronic stress makes itself felt. All those agitated hormones, swilling fats and tensed muscles haven't had a chance to go away. They've holed up in various corners of the body, waiting to pounce.

And when they do, they can cause:

★ Aches and pains, especially in the back and chest.
★ Heart palpitations.
★ Fainting, dizziness, sweating.
★ Twitching and trembling.
★ Stammering.
★ Indigestion and stomach aches.
★ Nausea.
★ Diarrhoea and frequency in urination.
★ Headaches.
★ Insomnia.
★ Breathlessness.
★ Hyperventilation (or overbreathing).
★ Choking sensations.
★ Loss of sexual libido.

I know I've overdrawn my bank balance of coping energy when a tiny muscle in the corner of my eye twitches uncontrollably, and I stammer when speaking to people. My husband gets indigestion; Geoffrey the banker has headaches and can't sleep. We all have our idiosyncratic warning signs.

Not only do our bodies protest, but our emotions and behaviour go all peculiar too. One of the earliest signs of overload is what Dr Chandra Patel, an expert in stress, calls 'an intensification of personality traits'. 'The suspicious person becomes defensive. The careful becomes over-meticulous, the pessimistic lugubrious, the anxious panic-stricken, the inadequate falls to pieces altogether. The irritable becomes explosive, the extrovert becomes slapdash and the introspective loses contact with everyday reality.'

Does that ring any bells?

If I'm tired I lose my appetite; other people say they have a compulsion to eat, snacking on fattening comfort foods.

Other emotional signs of fatigue are:

★ Depression.
★ Panic attacks.
★ Feeling exhausted and lethargic, even in the morning.
★ Drinking too much alcohol.
★ Smoking in excess.
★ Nail-biting.
★ Crying easily over 'nothing'.
★ Letting yourself go – not bothering to keep yourself or your home clean and attractive.
★ Lack of concentration.
★ Finding it hard to make decisions.
★ Memory lapses.
★ A lack of interest or enthusiasm in anything.
★ Inefficiency.
★ Anxiety.
★ Hypochondria – worrying about getting ill.
★ Phobias and obsessions (Let me share this with you: if I'm really worn out and stressed I can't leave the house without checking that all the electric plugs are switched off – aaargh.)

WHAT CAUSES STRESS?

When anyone mentions causes of stress (stressors), sooner or later the Holmes Rahe 'social readjustment rating scale' (happily renamed the Stress Chart) crops up. This allots stress points for various life events on a scale of one to 100, and if you tot them up for everything occurring to you in the last 12 months you can, in theory, work out your chances of developing a stress-related illness.

Devised as far back as the 1960s by two American psychologists, Dr Thomas Holmes and Dr Richard Rahe, it is utterly fascinating (even when you disagree with what can seem rather arbitrary ratings) and reassuring in a curious way. No wonder everyone had hysterics over our wedding, you think: getting married rates 50 points, which is three more than losing your job and eleven more than pregnancy. (But then Drs Holmes and Rahe have obviously never been pregnant.)

Anyway, here it is:

LIFE EVENTS	STRESS POINTS
Death of spouse	100
Divorce	73
Marital separation	65
Gaol sentence	63
Death of close family member	63
Personal injury or illness	53
Marriage/engagement/living together	50
Loss of job	47
Marital reconciliation	45
Retirement	45
Change in health of family member	44
Pregnancy	39
Sex difficulties	39
Birth of baby	39
Business readjustment	39
Change in financial state	38
Death of a close friend	37
Change to a different line of work	36
Change in number of arguments with spouse	35
Large mortgage or loan	31

Foreclosure of mortgage or loan	30
Change in responsibilities at work	29
Son or daughter leaving home	29
Trouble with in-laws	28
Outstanding personal achievement	28
Spouse/partner begins or stops work	26
Beginning or end of school or college	26
Change in living conditions	25
Revision of personal habits (more exercise, giving up smoking)	24
Trouble with the boss	23
Change in work hours or conditions	20
Change in residence/moving house	20
Change in school or college	20
Change in recreation	19
Change in church/social activities	19
Moderate mortgage or loan	18
Change in sleeping habits	17
Change in number of family gatherings	16
Change in eating habits, such as dieting	15
Holiday	13
Christmas	12
Minor violations of the law	11

A score of more than 300 indicates a serious life crisis – you could expect to be heavily affected. Between 150 and 299 you have a moderate chance of developing a stress-related illness, such as depression, and less than 150 – well, don't wait up.

Of course, this doesn't mean you *will* collapse in a gibbering heap by a long shot. 'Oh my God,' you may be crying, 'I've got married *and* moved house *and* had a baby *and* changed jobs *and* gone on holiday *and* taken out a large mortgage *and* won the London Marathon, and that's over 200 points and half of them weren't even *lousy* life events. What if something *really* nasty happens?'

There are people who draw on inner strength to endure the most appalling catastrophes, and others go down like a ninepin over relatively minor mishaps. How you survive stress – or rather, the events causing it – depends on a complex of factors. Your personality, for a start. Anxious people will worry themselves into a tizzy of sleeplessness and exhaustion over a problem that somebody else takes in their stride.

'It's all relative,' says my friend Sandra, who returned to full-time work in local government after raising a family. 'When I first went into the office, I was on tenterhooks. Of course, it didn't help that I was on six months trial, which was obligatory for every new employee, but I was so unaccustomed to the work and my colleagues were so new and strange, I felt that the slightest mistake would be a sacking offence and that everyone was judging me and passing comment. I worried myself sick over whether a letter was correctly phrased, or if I'd said the wrong thing at a meeting, and would come home shattered and collapse into bed.

'Two years later I just look back in astonishment. These days I never think twice about going into meetings, and the kind of incidents I'd be in turmoil over then float past with barely a ripple. I know the system and the people, what's important and what's not.'

How deeply and in what way a stressful event affects you is coloured by the context of your life. A chap who's been made redundant, whose wife is threatening to leave, whose children are truanting from school, whose home is about to be repossessed, will not, you must admit, be well placed to sail through a minor traffic infringement. Indeed, it could be the proverbial Last Straw, the final evidence that he is an incompetent human being who doesn't deserve another minute on this planet.

On the other hand, of course, it could pale into such insignificance beside his other catastrophes that he simply ignores it, fretting over it infinitely less than the conscientious driver alarmed at a blot on his immaculate record.

Reference

Which? Understanding Stress (Hodder & Stoughton)

THE MIND–BODY CONNECTION

Driven underground, stress can nibble away at the immune system with which the body repels disease. Recent research indicates that when you are under severe pressure, the antibodies and killer cells relied on to wipe out invading viruses and bacteria either can't do their jobs properly, or are unable to muster the necessary numbers. Marshalling your resources to deal with some of the obvious threats on your horizon seems to leave you vulnerable to other, less visible ones.

Losing your job, being burgled or experiencing a death in the family nearly doubles your risk of catching a cold, according to a study of 400 volunteers at the Medical Research Council's now defunct Common Cold Unit in Wiltshire. Your personality comes into it too. How you cope with both daily hassles and what scientists call 'major life events' – bereavement, divorce, redundancy – can determine your susceptibility to disease, say psychologists Julie Turner and Professor Andrew Steptoe of St George's Hospital, London.

The hyper-organised (and frequently exhausted) working mother rushing to keep to her schedule, dashing home to whip up supper and chivvy the children to piano practice and homework – an all-too-familiar picture of someone trying to keep all the balls in the air, in fact – is more likely to fall victim to a cold than the laid-back parent who leaves the plates unwashed while she reads a book with the kids.

And don't allow yourself the luxury of losing your temper,

snarling at your spouse or kicking the cat. You'll only increase the risk. Families low on conflict as well as organisation also reported fewer colds, says Julie Turner.

Blood samples from students at Ohio State University show that the number of killer cells, the immune system's crack troops in fighting infection, slumped during exams, a period of high stress and anxiety. And the lonelier the students, the fewer friends they had to support and distract them, then the bigger the drop. Other research indicates that introverts, who tend to be lonely people, are known to suffer more from viral infections: their colds are snufflier, their noses runnier.

Is there really a connection between the swirling emotions of the mind and the nuts and bolts, only-if-you-see-it-touch-it-can-it-exist world of the body? Intuitively we assume the two are intertwined and have done so for centuries: our language is full of expressions such as 'white with fear' and 'boiling with rage'. Exams give us butterflies in the tummy; pushy drivers and rude sales assistants are a pain in the neck. Smile, we say, and you'll feel better.

Doctors and scientists, however, are trained to see the world differently. They abide by what is called the Cartesian Dualism, the principle that has guided modern science since the 18th-century French philosopher Descartes kept the Pope happy by declaring mind and body were separate entities: the mind or soul belonging to the Church, the body to science, and never the twain shall meet.

According to Western medicine, we are composed of tangible, observable things such as atoms and molecules. Physical changes have physical causes, and you catch a cold because an aggressive virus has overwhelmed your antibodies, as simple as that. Eat oranges for vitamin C, take a paracetamol to dampen feverishness, go to bed early and avoid germ-laden people. How can something as nebulous as feelings, scientists ask scathingly, influence the cells of the immune system?

And yet evidence piles up to support the mind's influence on physical illness. Bereaved people, racked with grief, have a lower resistance to disease. Hostile individuals run a greater risk of heart disease. Those in stressful jobs where they have little personal control over their work are two to four times more likely to get sick.

Here is the good news: the mind has healing powers too. At Stanford University in California, breast cancer patients who formed strong bonds with each other in a support group lived twice as long as expected. In the UK, Dr Stephen Greer found that women with a fighting spirit or who refused to acknowledge their disease had a better chance of surviving breast cancer. Learning to be assertive and express emotions seems to improve melanoma patients' chances of living longer. Patients need less pain control if anaesthetists hold their hands and explain their surgery to them; they even recover more quickly if they can see trees from their hospital windows.

Now it appears there could be a physiological explanation that will satisfy sceptics. A pioneering American biochemist, Dr Candace Pert, claims that tiny proteins known as neuropeptides, produced by nerve and other cells, act as chemical messengers linking the brain and different systems of the body – and they are stimulated by our emotions.

How? Take endorphins, the brain's natural pain-relievers that lie behind emotional experiences such as the runner's 'high' and the lover's orgasm. These are also neuropeptides and have recently been discovered not only in the brain, but in the immune system too. In theory, we can register emotion in every part of our body, even our big toe. Mind and body, says Dr Pert, are inextricably linked as one organism. What affects one will immediately impact on the other. The shopkeeper is rude, you are angry; you run into a friend and feel pleasure; she tells you her mother is ill and you are sad and sympathetic. As our emotions fluctuate, so the body mixes different cocktails of peptides, constantly changing and adjusting. Waves of subtle signals sweep up and down our bodies, causing muscles to tense and relax, blood pressure to rise and fall.

That's the hypothesis. The challenge now is to discover which

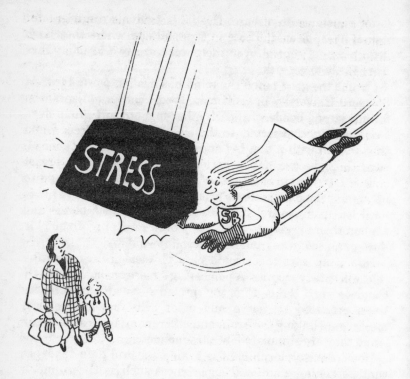

emotion is tied to which neuropeptide – and then how to summon it up when needed.

But what does all this have to do with fatigue and stress?

For a start, it's a serious argument that you can do something about feeling tired all the time. By changing how you behave and feel about what's happening in your life, you could influence, even liberate, your physical sources of energy and well-being. Dr Pert believes that it is vital that we release our emotions, allowing strong feelings such as grief, sorrow, anger and fear to be expressed. Hanging onto them is tiring, and locks up energy that could be put to better use. 'Part of being a healthy person is being well integrated and at peace, with all the systems acting together,' she says.

90

Of course we can't do it all by ourselves, nor should we fall into the trap of taking too much responsibility for our state of health – the 'if I get sick it's my fault because I didn't try hard enough' syndrome. ('If I had all the answers to that, I wouldn't be trying to lose my 30 pounds in excess weight,' says Candace Pert crisply. 'I'd simply call up my peptides and get myself into a state of mind where I hate food and want to exercise.')

It's more about learning how to mobilise our resources to give ourselves the best possible chance. At a basic level, it means nurturing our bodies – eating well and keeping fit – but on another, the intellectual and emotional level, it means opening our minds to new ideas, new therapies, new strategies; learning to trust other people, perhaps, or listening to inner voices that we've ignored for years.

Yes, it's a little scary. Once you start lifting the lid who knows what will come crawling out, or where it will stop? But not all change has to be radical. Sure, some people might discover they want to chuck in their jobs and take off for chicken farming in the Hebrides – but something as simple as a regular aromatherapy massage, or a dinner with friends once a week, could invigorate your life, and introduce a dimension and enthusiasm that you had thought impossible.

The question is – where to begin?

CHAPTER 7

What you can do immediately . . .

INSTANT RELIEF

. . .Well, in the next 24 hours.

A simple change in routine could be enough to break the fatigue cycle. At the very least, it could refresh you enough to keep going, or allow you sufficient space to think about what to do in the long term. It's even possible to learn how to re-energise (shades of *Star Trek*) without leaving your chair.

Take five

This exercise is so low key you can do it at your office desk, and your colleagues will hardly notice. Begin by making sure the chair supports your back and neck. Put your hands on your lap and close your eyes. Breathe gently and rhythmically, feeling your stomach move in and out. Starting with your feet and working upwards, note where any tension is in your body, and puff it away with each outward breath. Drop your head forward but keep it straight, as though a string on the crown of your head ran towards the ceiling. When you feel warm and relaxed, think of something agreeable – walking by a stream, perhaps, or lying on a sunny beach. Even five minutes of this will perk you up, but stay with it if you can for fifteen.

Go AWOL

Imagine dropping out, walking away from it all. Leave the report half-written, committee members at each other's throats, the fridge empty of food, and one hundred and one pieces of Lego on the living room floor. Where, in fantasy, would you like to be?

I take myself out to Heathrow airport and board a jet for the Great Barrier Reef. There's an island there where the sand curves gently into a limpid sea, and fish of emerald green, of cobalt blue and citron yellow dart between coral fringes. And in the evening you sip a long iced punch beneath the palm trees and watch a tropic sun sink in a tumescence of gold.

Call it daydreaming if you prefer. Stress management therapists use the technique with overwrought clients who are spinning so fast they threaten to whizz wildly off into the stratosphere. Just close your eyes and walk out, mentally, on everything.

Picture it. Your secretary fielding the telephone calls – 'no, unavailable, I'm afraid.' Your boss unable to chair the meeting because you haven't briefed her. At home, the family staring at each other in stupefaction over empty plates. Instead of straining at the leash to escape the moment you walk in the door, the nanny will have to stay late. Tsk. Gas bills won't be paid. The lawn will be un-mown. The cat won't be fed.

And where are you? In Florence, perhaps, on the art appreciation course you've always yearned to do. Hiking over the Cairngorms. Maybe just round the corner, lying in the sun on the grass by the river. And curiously, surprisingly, in your absence the world manages to stumble on. Instead of leaving all the dreary research work to you, your boss has to buckle down and find out a few facts for herself. Your partner discovers the location of the supermarket. The children put themselves to bed. The cat miaows so hideously somebody gives it dinner.

You'll be missed, of course – but it might just help put some things in perspective. Are you the only one in the family capable of doing the shopping? Is your employer taking you just a tad too much for granted? Why are you always the one carting home extra work? Maybe the fundraising committee deserves to sink if you're the only one propping it up. And will life as you know it *really* collapse if the kitchen floor isn't swept once a day?

Dump the chores
Nothing is more fatiguing or dispiriting to most women than
a messy, dirty house – especially if the mess and the dirt
have been generated by others than yourself. Nagging them
into cleaning it up is even more exhausting – teenagers are
notoriously deaf to pleas, and blind to the kind of squalor
that would offend a sewer rat. If you can't see the walls for
the rubbish, call in a cleaning company for a one-off purge –
or consider a cleaning woman on a regular basis. The boost to
your spirits might justify the expense, and free you to earn
the fee.

'Picking up the odd meal from M&S changed my life,' says
Lottie, a physiotherapist with two children under ten and a
husband rarely home before seven thirty. 'At first I felt guilty –
spending money on prepared food and not playing earth mother
over the stove every night – but what I gain in extra energy
and patience for the kids after a hectic day is worth every
penny.'

Go for a walk
Get out in the fresh air and feel your limbs moving. You're not
hurrying to catch a train, just walking. Head for a park or
green spaces. Clear your head of worries and let the trees and
grass and people flow by you.

Stre-e-e-tch
Clare Maxwell-Hudson, Britain's leading massage therapist,
recommends these simple stretches to relieve fatigue-causing
muscle tension:

1. Link your hands together behind your back and, whilst
    straightening your arms, try to bring your elbows
    together. Hold the stretch for fifteen seconds. Repeat
    twice.
2. With your hands still linked behind your back, your feet
    hip width apart, stretch your arms up as far back as they
    will go. Breathe out and bend forward at the hips. Let

your arms come up over your head. Hold for a count of
fifteen. Repeat. This should be a relaxing pose to increase
flexibility.

3. In the same position but now with your hands resting
    on your hips at your lower back, press your hands on
    your hips to give your lower back a gentle stretch.
    Repeat.

4. Now link your hands again, this time putting them above
    your head with the palms facing upwards. Push your
    arms slightly up and back. Hold the stretch for fifteen
    seconds. Relax.

Remember to keep your breathing deep and rhythmic,
and remain as relaxed as possible.

Take a bath
Run a warm bath, add six to ten drops of a stimulating
essential oil and wallow in the water for at least ten minutes.
Or add a few drops to a tissue and sniff. Revitalising oils
include:

Rosemary – good for mental and physical exhaustion. Ancient
Greeks are said to have worn garlands of rosemary when
taking examinations. (Avoid rosemary if you are pregnant,
however – it could be *too* stimulating.)
Basil – clears a jaded mind after intense concentration.
Bergamot – uplifting when you feel worn out and down.
Sandalwood – gives an energising boost.

Take a fizzy bath to spark up tired tissues. Add a few spoonfuls
of bicarbonate of soda so the water bubbles refreshingly against
your skin.

Freshen up with a shower
A quick and easy pick-me-up. Keep the temperature coolish,
brush your body with a loofah, and turn the tap to cold before
stepping out.

Skin brush
Do this before stepping into the bath or shower. When pores become choked with old skin cells, it's harder for the body to rid itself of waste products. Skin brushing also improves blood and lymph circulation, one reason it feels so invigorating.

Use a dry, firm brush – a dry loofah will do, but a special brush is available – and brush very gently at first, gradually increasing the pressure over the next few days. Start at the soles of your feet and work your way up your legs, your front and your back. Then do your hands and up your arms. Focus the brush strokes, when doing your chest and upper back, towards your heart. Miss out your face, but give the back of your neck and scalp a good go.

Dry Skin Brush available from Green Farm Catalogue,
225 Putney Bridge Road,
London SW15 2PY
(tel. 081-874 1130)

Make an appointment for a massage or facial
A massage can be either soothing or invigorating (or both) and a brisk, light general massage is great at renewing frayed body systems. Even more blissful is aromatherapy, as the essential oils used are absorbed by the skin and carried round the body in the bloodstream for maximum effect. Make sure that you tell the aromatherapist why you want the massage so she chooses the most appropriate oils. You'll smell glorious and benefits are claimed to last days and even weeks.

Find your pressure points
This is an amazingly simple technique that you can perform in the middle of a meeting and nobody will be any the wiser. Acupressure is like acupuncture but you use your fingers instead of needles. According to traditional Chinese medicine, healing energy (Qi) flows along pathways in the body known as meridians, and enters and exits at various points at skin level.

Pressure on these points can clear any blockages affecting health.

Acupoints to relieve fatigue are:

1. At the centre of the palm at the point where the middle finger rests when folded inwards.
2. In the middle section of the little finger.

    Press firmly on the acupoint with the tips of your fingers or the ball of your thumb, and increase pressure gradually until you reach a weight of about five grams (practise on the kitchen scales). Hold this for 20 seconds and then release gently. Wait ten seconds and repeat the process five times.

Plan a weekend away

'It can be hard to switch off when you're too close to your working life,' says Tom, a trade magazine editor. 'We used to have a country cottage where we vegged out at weekends, and it was a real lifesaver on occasion. A hundred miles out of London, nobody in the village cared about my job. I could sleep in without a nagging feeling I should be reading papers or mowing the lawn or any of the hundred and one things you feel obliged to do at home. And in the afternoon you walked through meadows with trees and cows, and the office felt a million miles away. Joy.

'We sold the cottage when the recession struck, but I've made it a rule to get away at least once a month. We stay at a bed and breakfast or a little country house hotel, forget about whatever happens on Monday to Friday, and drive back to London on Sunday evening feeling as if we've been away for a week.'

Escaping from home with its constant reminders of daily pressures – your briefcase in the hall, shirts to wash, the pile of unread journals, the uncut hedge – is a chance to stand outside yourself and forget everything for a couple of days; just long enough to be a tonic and allow you an emotional as well as physical breath of fresh air.

Treat yourself to a health farm

If you're going away to unwind and revitalise, consider putting yourself in the hands of experts. Yes, it is horribly expensive, but justifiable if you're at the end of your tether. Health farms are shamelessly dedicated to pampering and restoring you, and you will have nothing more taxing to do than remember your massage appointment, or where to find the sauna. People slop about in track suits and towelling robes and put their brains on ice. It's a wonderful opportunity to try out exotic treatments such as reflexology and hydrotherapy and the food, contrary to mythology, is ample and wholesomely delicious.

Take a nap

Oh yeah, you say, in the middle of the day? Why not? It's not as silly as it sounds. Winston Churchill won World War II on the strength of his cat naps – fifteen minutes or so when he switched off for a restorative doze. 'Ten minutes after lunch is worth an hour at night,' a high-living aunt would declare, disappearing into her bedroom as soon as the Sunday roast had cleared the table.

After lunch is an excellent time to start practising the habit, when the post-prandial dip in energy makes concentration difficult and there's a natural sagging of spirits. It might prove something of an acquired skill, especially if you're one to scorn flopping on beds once you're up and dressed, but you don't have to actually get back between the sheets. Lie on the sofa, if you feel happier, and put a newspaper over your face.

Childbirth relaxation classes during my first pregnancy taught me both the knack and the benefits of The Nap (see page 106 for Learn to Relax). By midday when my brain felt like jelly and my limbs like sandbags, I'd lie on the bed, close my eyes, do as the instructor said and imagine myself heavy as lead, sinking into a black velvet curtain, and bingo, twenty minutes later I'd be coming to, fresh as the proverbial daisy. Once the baby was born, one was so exhausted with changing nappies, feeding and winding and walking up and down that the moment the infant went to sleep, I'd seize the opportunity to do the same. And by the time it trotted off to playschool, I was adept at grabbing the odd ten or twenty minutes for a snooze.

Nowadays, if I'm planning to work late in the evening I find an after-lunch nap clears my head and gives me the energy to make the most of those extra hours. But that's the advantage of working at home, you'll be saying crossly. What about those of us stuck in the middle of an office or behind a counter?

Well, there *is* Saturday and Sunday. A nap on two days out of seven isn't a bad start, and will help you recuperate from a heavy week. A friend who works fiendishly hard in public relations, with meetings, business lunches and often evening engagements crammed into her timetable, makes a point of lying down with an airline mask over her eyes as soon as she steps through her door after work. 'Twenty minutes,' she says, 'and I'm a new woman.'

Twenty minutes, incidentally, appears to be the magic time for the perfect nap. Much longer and you go into a deeper sleep, from which it's difficult to recover and function effectively. Set the alarm if you're afraid you'll go over, but with practice, you can train yourself to surface at just the right moment.

Even if you can't curl up on a couch, your office might be quiet or private enough to let you put your head down on the desk during lunch hour. On summer days, too, city parks are littered with workers dozing in the sunshine. Why not join them?

Get a good night's sleep

Easier said than done – especially when insomnia is a major contributor to your fatigue. If only I *could* sleep, you moan; then I wouldn't feel so lethargic and zonked out during the day. I'd concentrate better and I wouldn't feel everything was getting on top of me.

Others can sleep all right – when they get the opportunity. Mothers with young children know all too well the dreadful drained feeling of night after night of interrupted sleep, coupled with the brain fatigue of a new routine and responsibilities. For businessmen and women, overwhelming work-

99

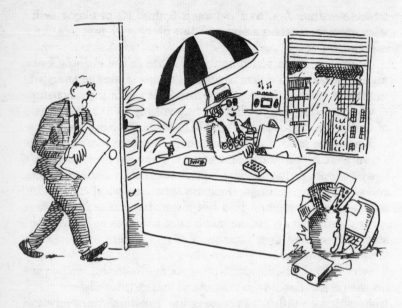

loads, long commutes and company travel mean skimped sleep, consistently getting by with an hour or two less than they need. Their sleep patterns are all over the place: one night they're up until 2 a.m., the next they're trying to nod off at ten because they have a 6 a.m. plane to catch in the morning. 'It's only when I get right away, on holiday or a long weekend in the country, that I enjoy the kind of sleep from which you wake really refreshed,' says a high-profile television executive.

We all know that a good night's sleep, when you wake bright and full of zest, conscious of having drunk deep of the elixir of life, can turn your world around. The impossible becomes achievable. Solutions to intractable problems suddenly appear. Despair turns to hope, irritation to tolerance. And yet sometimes the more we yearn for such sleep, the more elusive it becomes.

Half of those Britons aged between 40 and 55 have occasional problems with sleep, and between 5 and 10 per cent will suffer enough to see a doctor. 'The killer is when you start observing yourself, wondering *how* you fall asleep,' complains an accomplished insomniac. But if you are one of those who lie wide-eyed at night, fruitlessly tossing and turning as you recycle the day's worries and the long small hours drag by, what can you do?

Here's a surprise: You might actually be getting as much sleep as you need. Researchers in sleep laboratories have discovered that many insomniacs are unaware when they are asleep. At Stanford University, California, doctors found that a 61-year-old college professor who had always regarded himself as an insomniac actually averaged eight hours' sleep a night. He stopped worrying as a result, found he woke less in the night, felt less depressed and less tired.

Perceptions of sleep differ too. Two people may each take half an hour to fall asleep and wake six hours later. One will complain of insomnia, the other claim to be a good sleeper.

We need sleep to rest and restore the brain, and the deepest, or delta, level of sleep, when the brain waves are long and flat, is the most refreshing of all. But don't keep yourself awake worrying about getting enough for your health. Your brain might feel a mite fuzzy, but physically you can survive for days without sleep, provided you get rest and adequate food. Relax and leave the problem to your body – when it needs sleep, it will take it.

It's another myth that we all need eight hours' sleep a night. Some of us – Margaret Thatcher is a classic example – operate very nicely thank you on four hours a night. Others are fine with six or seven. Six hours, according to Professor Jim Horne, who runs the sleep laboratory at Loughborough University and is a leading authority on insomnia, is usually enough to avoid daytime sleepiness. If you still feel drained and fatigued, he says, it's usually not sleepiness that's the problem but weariness and exhaustion associated with depression or chronic stress. Treat these underlying problems and the insomnia will disappear.

People complaining of sleeplessness fall into three categories: those who can't go to sleep; those who fall asleep but wake frequently during the night; and those who wake early in the morning and can't go back to sleep again. Early waking is often associated with stress and depression. In severe cases, a doctor may prescribe antidepressants.

Sleeping pills have their place, but preferably in the short term. A marketing manager who makes frequent flights to Hong Kong and Australia is one of many travellers who resort to temazepam, a short-acting cousin of diazepam (Valium) that allows four and a half hours of sound sleep. 'It knocks you out on a long-haul flight, and helps you readjust your sleep pattern the night you arrive,' he says. During the Gulf War, when aircrews flew punishing hours, with as little as six hours between one period of duty and the next, it was temazepam that kept them going and helped prevent the disastrous 'microsleeps' that over-worked doctors and lorry drivers have reported.

For chronic insomniacs, doctors are turning to more ingenious, and ultimately natural methods, than zapping them with pills. Sleep restriction therapy is currently top of the pops. Instead of going to bed, you're ordered to stay up.

Philip, a 28-year-old accountant who'd wrestled with sleeplessness for six months, was told not to go to bed before midnight, to set his alarm for 6 a.m. and get up when it went off, no matter how exhausted he felt. Daytime naps and weekend lie-ins were out, because they make an insomniac less sleepy at night. And if he wasn't asleep in ten minutes, he must get up and do something else until he felt sleepy again.

Philip says the cure worked like a charm. There were several nights and days of shattering fatigue, but a month later he was sleeping better than ever, and the doctor was allowing him to go to bed fifteen minutes earlier. Eventually he settled on a period of sleep that enabled him to feel rested without beginning to lie awake.

Reference

Sleep Matters (support group for insomniacs),
  10 Barley Mow Passage,
  Chiswick,
  London W4 4PH
  (tel. 081-994 6477)

Drop-off tips

★ Keep off caffeine, preferably from midday onwards. Coffee is the major villain, but remember there is caffeine in tea (a cuppa before bedtime is *not* a good idea), chocolate, and some pain relievers.

★ Avoid alcohol. It may help you nod off, but can prevent a deep sleep, and could wake you later in the night.

★ Don't smoke. Nicotine raises the blood pressure and pulse rate.

★ Don't eat a large meal within two and preferably three hours of going to bed. Your stomach will be working hard to digest it, a difficult job at the end of the day.

★ A bedtime snack is okay – especially if it's a sleep-promoting food with high levels of the amino acid tryptophan, which helps produce calming serotonin in the brain. Milk, bananas, tuna, eggs, poultry, cheese, and pasta are all loaded with tryptophan, which works even more effectively if combined with carbohydrates. The old nursery remedy of a cup of hot milk and wholemeal biscuit really does the trick.

★ Herbal remedies have been tried and tested over centuries, and are now easily available in tablet form from health-food shops and chemists. Valerian is an ancient sleeping potion (beware taking high doses over a long period, however – it has been associated with liver failure). Other people swear by hop pillows and by lavender and camomile – both as teas and essential oils for the bath or pillow.

★ Get some exercise during the day to relieve stress hormones – but avoid anything too strenuous within three hours before bedtime.

★ The exception to the above is sex! Good lovemaking relaxes the body and mind.

★ Try to keep regular bedtime hours. Raving on Saturday night and sleeping in on Sunday morning sets your body clock back a couple of hours, creating what researchers call 'Sunday night insomnia'.

★ Make sure your bedroom is calm and comfortable. Some people like a bed with a firm mattress, but go with whatever feels good for you. Avoid temperature extremes – in the dream phase of sleep, your body can't regulate temperature by sweating or shivering. Over 75°F and sleep is disturbed.

★ Put worries out of your mind (if you can) and avoid arguments after supper.

★ Practise relaxation and visualisation exercises to release tension:

– Lie on your back, arms by your sides, eyes closed and imagine yourself so heavy you are sinking through the floor. Tense and then relax muscles from the toes upwards. Breathe gently and rhythmically, slowly withdrawing your mind from your surroundings.

– Picture yourself somewhere soothing, in a meadow perhaps or by the sea, and breathe deeply, imagining the soft sigh of a breeze or the lull of water.

– Count backwards from 100 (you can forget the sheep!), allowing your body to relax a little more with each number.

– Breathe deeply and evenly and repeat a comforting word or phrase, such as 'peace'.

★ If you're still wide awake fifteen minutes after getting into bed, don't lie there fretting. Get up, go into another room so that your bedroom is not associated with worry, and do something else – read, watch television, sip warm milk – until you feel sleepy.

★ If you wake early with the dawn light in summer, invest in heavier curtains or wear a sleeping mask to bed. Better to look like the Lone Ranger than a zombie.

Check out how well you cope with stress
Do you:

1. Take at least one hot, balanced meal per day?
2. Have seven hours' sleep at least four nights a week?
3. Give and receive affection frequently?
4. Have a relative within 50 miles on whom you can rely?
5. Exercise to perspiration at least twice per week?
6. Smoke less than ten cigarettes per day?
7. Take alcohol less than five times a week?
8. Keep within the appropriate weight for your height?
9. Have an adequate income for your needs?
10. Get strength from religious, philosophical or some other deeply held beliefs?
11. Regularly attend a social evening?
12. Have a network of friends and acquaintances?
13. Have a close friend to confide in?
14. Enjoy good health?
15. Express feelings of anger or worry?
16. Have regular domestic discussions (*not* arguments) with those you live with?
17. Do something for fun at least once a week?
18. Organise your time effectively?
19. Drink less than three cups of caffeine (tea, coffee or cola) a day?
20. Have a quiet time to yourself each day?

Score one point for *yes/always*; two points for *probably/usually*; three points for *I suppose/it depends*; four points for *rarely/not a lot*; five points for *no/never*.
If your score adds up to less than 50 you probably cope well with stress. Higher scores indicate an increasing vulnerability in stressful situations.
(Adapted from a questionnaire devised by Lyle H. Miller and Alma Dill Smith of Boston University Medical Center, USA.)

Learn to relax
This is a deep muscle relaxation technique to help you unwind, focus on your inner self and release the muscle tension that causes fatigue. Use it, too, to send yourself to sleep.

1. Wear loose comfortable clothes and make sure your feet are warm. Being furthest from your heart they will be the first to feel cold.

2. Ensure the room is warm, dark and quiet and that you won't be disturbed for at least a quarter of an hour. Lock the door. Tell the children to watch television. Then lie down on the floor, on a mat or a firm mattress, with a rug over you if you think the room could get chilly. As you relax, your body temperature will drop. Place a cushion under your head and knees. Let your hands and arms rest by your side, palms upwards.

3. Relax and take a couple of deep, sighing breaths. Empty your mind.

4. One by one, tense and let go all the muscles in your body, beginning with the toes, then the feet, calves, knees, buttocks, stomach, working gradually up the body until you end with the face. Tighten and release first one leg then the other; one arm then the other. As you let go feel how warm and heavy the muscles are, how they sink into the floor. Your limbs should feel numb and impossible to move.

5. Hunch your shoulders towards your ears, then let go, letting them sink into the floor.

6. Rock your head gently to loosen your neck.

7. Begin to relax the face with a yawn. Let go. Purse the lips and let go. Frown then relax. Raise your eyebrows, then let go.

8. By now you should feel so buried in the floor that you can't bear to move. Breathe in and out evenly. On each outward breath tell yourself you are more relaxed, more peaceful . . .

9. Remain thus for fifteen minutes. (You might even go to

106

sleep.) Set a timer if necessary.
10. When it's time to return to the rat race, open your eyes gradually. Turn on your side, then slowly, gently bring yourself to a sitting position and get up.

Reference

The Complete Book of Relaxation Techniques by Jenny Sutcliffe (Headline)

CHAPTER 8

Eating for energy

YOU ARE WHAT YOU EAT *OR* FOOD, GLORIOUS FOOD?

Our bodies, like motor cars, run on fuel. They need filling up regularly, and they perform better on the right kind of stuff. There, I suppose, the analogy ends – with the exception of a breed of young men whose automobile is a curious extension of themselves, and who would probably spend more on its maintenance than they would on their own. You need only see them polishing their gleaming megahorsepower chariots one moment and the next pushing junk food down their throats – greasy chips, fat-sodden polystyrene hamburgers and sugar-stuffed chocolate bars – to be convinced of this.

It *should* be blindingly obvious that if you don't eat appropriate food in adequate amounts you are not going to function as well as you should. If, for instance, you skimp breakfast because you're late (a cup of coffee) then rush lunch because you want to go shopping (a lukewarm slab of salami pizza at a snack bar), eke out the afternoon with a chocolate biscuit, and after work put away two glasses of wine, a packet of crisps, a slice of soggy quiche and a cappuccino coffee, then you haven't exactly consumed the optimum daily requirements of carbohydrate, protein, fat, vitamins and minerals. And if you keep up this haphazard diet for one reason or another – you have a disorganised desire to lose weight, you forget to visit the supermarket, you're up to your ears with work and can't think about food – then sooner or later something is going to give.

When we lack enough nutrients to create the energy that powers our body systems, our muscles tire, our brain flags, and our immune defences pack up. We feel exhausted, miserable, depressed, and every beastly virus that happens along has its wicked way with us.

'But I take a multivitamin/ginseng/kelp/garlic pill/evening primrose oil/whatever,' I hear you cry. Well, yes – and they have their role – but you can't expect supplements to *take the place* of food. In fact, some experts believe that taking a vitamin or a mineral on its own may not always be as effective as when they are in a food 'package' with other nutrients.

But then the whole food supplement issue is racked with controversy. Nutrition has the power to arouse more passions, more myths and fads and confusion than almost anything else to do with health.

For years we've been bombarded with conflicting advice. Margarine is good for you because butter is full of fat which blocks up arteries. Margarine is not so good for you because too much polyunsaturated fat might cause cancer. Don't eat potatoes because they are fattening and full of starch. Eat potatoes because they are full of starch and starch is now good for you. Use olive oil because it protects against heart disease. Whoops, not so sure about that, so go easy on the olive oil. Don't eat nuts because they are full of calories. Eat nuts because they are full of vitamin E.

Fortunately, international nutritionists have at last settled on a few simple rules for a healthy diet. This wisdom can be summed up in three sentences:

1. Half your diet should be starchy food such as bread, pasta, rice or potatoes.
2. Eat at least five portions of fruit and vegetables a day.
3. Eat as little as possible of saturated fat.

If you like facts served in little mental pictures, imagine a pyramid divided into three layers. At the base, the largest layer that should also comprise the largest part of your diet, are vegetables, fruit, pulses (beans and lentils), cereal and bread. In the middle layer, to be eaten in moderation, are milk, cheese, yoghurt, lean meat, poultry, fish, nuts and eggs. Finally, at the apex, for least consumption of all, are sugar, butter, margarine and oil.

As a mother who's supposed to prepare nutritious wholesome meals for a grateful family, I've found the easiest way to get to grips with this concept is to discard the old idea of a good meal as meat and two veg. Think instead 'will it be bread, potatoes, rice or pasta tonight?' and construct the menu accordingly.

Why are starchy foods important?
Starchy foods, or carbohydrates, are our fastest source of energy. The body transforms them to glucose, the main sugar in the blood and the body's basic fuel.

There are two main types: the 'good' or complex carbohydrates, and the 'not so good', the simple carbohydrates or sugars.

Complex carbohydrates include: bread, rice, pasta, potatoes, pulses, whole grains, other cereals, and root vegetables such as sweet potatoes. They are better for you because they carry lots of nutritional extras, such as dietary fibre, vitamins and minerals, *and* – despite their previous bad press – they are not fattening. It's not the potatoes in potato chips that stack on the calories; it's the oil in which they're drenched.

Sugars turn up in – apart from the sugar bowl – cakes, biscuits, pastries, honey, concentrated fruit juices, and as glucose syrup. Read the labels on processed and tinned foods and you'll be astonished at the amounts of sugar added to products like ham and soups. Sweet manufacturers love talking about 'pure food energy' but, compared to complex carbohydrates, it's an empty package – nothing but calories.

Two slices of wholemeal bread might contain 130 calories, compared with 130 in 330 mls of cola. But look what you get with the bread: five grams of protein, 1.5 grams of fat, plus the B vitamins riboflavin, thiamine and niacin, calcium, iron *and* fibre. The soft drink has zilch.

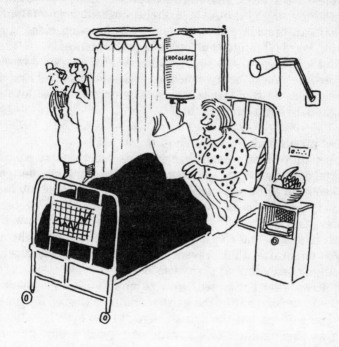

Can sugar deliver a quick energy punch?

It's tempting to regard carbohydrates as an instant energy
boost – especially sugar. Loads of people are convinced that a
sugary snack before an athletic event will give them a surge
of superpower (and justify a tasty piece of chocolate), but it
can actually work the other way. Sugar *will* raise glucose
levels and provide energy temporarily, but the insulin
released drags glucose levels even lower than they were to
start with. If taken before a long workout, it can actually
exhaust you faster, because your body has to call on its
energy reserves (glycogen stored in the liver and muscles)
earlier than usual.

So why do marathon runners graze on well-known snack bar

111

brands? As always, there are exceptions. Eating or drinking something sugary during an exercise workout *longer than two hours* can provide additional energy to keep up blood sugar levels, ward off fatigue and enhance performance.

But – in general – if you want short-term energy, a bowl of sugar-free muesli or a wholemeal roll – both full of complex carbohydrates that cause less seesawing of glucose levels – might deliver a better result.

How much fruit and veg should you eat?

A diet that helps prevent heart disease, diet-related cancers, dental decay, arthritis, osteoporosis and obesity is also designed to keep you as fit and energetic as possible. So when nutritionists say eat 14 ounces – or five portions – of fruit and vegetables a day, they mean it. It's an excellent source of fibre, as well as carbohydrates and the magic micronutrients – vitamins and trace minerals – that prevent fatigue. Don't include potatoes though; these count as starchy food.

I accept that I'm biased, growing up in a country where we picked passion fruit in the garden and breakfasted on papaya and pineapples, but the British haven't been exactly outstanding at loading their tables with sexy plant foods. In many households *even now*, an apple or an orange is about as exciting as you get, and the poor old cabbage and carrots and greens have been boiled until mushy and any goodness went down the sink with the cooking water.

But tastes are changing, and supermarkets now boast positively exotic ranges of tropical fruit and salad vegetables. (That much of it is rock solid and tasteless from refrigerated transport should not be cavilled at – one does get the occasional ripe avocado.) Mediterranean and Eastern cuisines have introduced ways of cooking – steaming and stir frying – that keep vegetables crisp and full of natural nutrients. One is permitted to crunch a carrot in the mouth nowadays.

But still – five portions of fruit and vegetables? Nearly a pound? A day? Don't panic. It's perfectly possible.

Try this arrangement:

Portion 1:   Fruit juice for breakfast.
Portion 2:   An apple, an orange or other piece of fruit mid-morning or afternoon.
Portion 3:   A fruit-based pudding – melon, apricots, peaches – after a meal.
Portions 4 and 5:   Two vegetables (other than potatoes) at the main meal.

There. Not too bad, really. And we could have squeezed in a few more. Be warned though – some fruit and vegetables carry more weight than others. You have to eat *sixteen* leaves of lettuce or *ten* brussels sprouts to equal two tablespoons of carrots, or two spears of broccoli.

What about protein?
What about it? Most meat-eaters probably get too much, and with saturated fats chucked in as well. My mother, being a good Australian, was a firm believer in meat as a source of strength and energy. 'It's full of protein,' she would say over the steak she liked to serve us for breakfast on examination days, usually with a couple of fried eggs winking on top as we tottered downstairs grey-faced from a night's cramming. 'You'll need it to get through the exam.'

The body needs protein to make muscles, organs, bones, skin, antibodies, some hormones and all enzymes, and it comes in the form of amino acids. Without these, our bodies would grind to a halt. Generally speaking, as long as we eat enough calories, we get enough protein. It's not stored, so a fresh supply is needed every day, to be shuffled into whichever amino acid building block the body needs at that moment.

There are nine 'essential' amino acids that we can't manufacture in our bodies and which we have to absorb directly by eating plants, or animals which consume plants.

Lysine, phenylalanine and tryptophan are at least three that you might encounter as over-the-counter health supplements. This is because most fruits, grains and vegetables lack one or more of the essential amino acids, and vegetarians therefore have to be careful to combine different foods so that they get the full whack – an even more challenging task for macrobiotic vegans. Meat and other animal products, such as cheese, eggs and milk, contain the lot, so eating them is the easiest way for most people to make sure they get sufficient protein.

There's no point eating more protein than you need, however, because it's not stored in the body and won't stimulate muscle growth or extra strength or endurance or anything else superhuman. Bodybuilders who throw T-bone steaks down their gullets aren't really achieving anything. Any excess is burned off as energy or converted to fat.

Are fats all bad?
Hmmmm, well . . . We need *some* fat to remain healthy. The question is how much and what kind.

We need fats in the body to store energy; to keep our skin and hair healthy; to carry the important fat-soluble vitamins A, D, E and K; and to supply the vital **essential fatty acids** (EFAs) that the body can't make – such as linoleic acid, important for growth. Fats actually *regulate* the amount of cholesterol in the blood, and, because they slow down food leaving the stomach, make us feel full and stop us eating too much.

Well, in theory.

There are two kinds of fat: *saturated*, which is found mainly in meat, milk and cheese, and *unsaturated*.

*Mono*unsaturated fats, as in olive oil, are the current heroes. It seems they can actually decrease cholesterol in the blood, and might *possibly* reduce the risk of heart disease.

*Poly*unsaturated fats (corn, safflower and sesame oils) were flavour of the month because they lowered the 'bad' (LDL) cholesterol that caused heart disease. Now, because they apparently also lower the 'good' (HDL) cholesterol, they've rather lost their gloss. Fish oil, though, is wonderful because it helps keep blood clotting in balance.

Why are fat people tired people?
Eat too much fat – of any kind – and you will get fat. It's not the sugar in cakes and pastries that puts on the pounds as much as the butter and oil.

Overweight and obese people suffer from fatigue because they are carrying too much weight around, putting excessive strain on their heart and other organs. You too would be tired if you were humping the equivalent of a small child or even a young adult around with you all the time. Yet one third of people in Western societies are overweight by 20 per cent. A very few of these may suffer from thyroid imbalances and other problems, but the vast majority are fat because they eat not too many calories so much as too many fats – and especially saturated fats.

Fat contains twice as many calories as protein or carbohydrate, and it's much easier to overindulge on fatty foods. Calories provide energy to keep our bodies ticking over, but what happens if we take too many on board? They settle around the tummy and thighs and other places as unlovely rolls of lard.

Exercise can work off excess calories, but fat people avoid strenuous activity. Whether this is *why* they are obese, or *because* they are obese, is difficult to tell.

The University of California, Berkeley, recommends the following strategies to lose weight:

★ Eat slowly.
★ Clear the fridge and pantry of high-calorie foods. Stock only what you intend to eat on your new diet.
★ Eat less fat and more complex carbohydrates.
★ Limit your intake of butter, ice cream, cheese, salad dressings and oils.
★ Avoid packaged snacks, biscuits and pastries.
★ Use nonstick pans and saucepans (less fat is needed in cooking).
★ Bake, grill or poach meats and steam vegetables. Don't fry.
★ Switch to skim milk and low fat dairy products.
★ Exercise regularly.

★ Take up activities that don't involve food – such as gardening.

★ Get counselling or join a support group such as Weight Watchers.

Aren't there any little magic energy pills?

Nutritionists insist until they are blue in the face that if your diet is well balanced and you get sufficient exercise, there is no need for additional vitamins and minerals. Everything that you require for good health should be in your food.

But does everyone eat a well-balanced diet? If you're tired and stressed, the first thing that can slip is sensible eating habits – a Catch 22 situation, because an insufficient supply of vitamins and minerals will only exacerbate your fatigue and feelings of inadequacy. A slippery slope, indeed.

'When I come home exhausted and irritable – which is most nights of the week – then I can't be bothered cooking a proper meal,' admits Vicky, a comprehensive school history teacher who lives alone. 'It'll be eggs or a piece of toast and cheese; something fast and easy. Rarely vegetables because I haven't got the energy to wash and cook them. Salads need messing about with, and lettuces and things tend to hang about the fridge rather too long – or at least mine do. I sometimes stick one of those ready-made meals in the microwave, but they usually come without veggies. It's pathetic, but we're under such an appalling workload that I just haven't got the time.'

'I smoke, I drink about six cups of coffee a day, and I'll have several pints of beer and the best part of a bottle of wine a day,' says Lloyd. 'Bad habits, I know, but there's too much aggro at work at the moment and this is the only way I know how to cope.'

Certain groups of people are also especially vulnerable to vitamin and mineral deficiencies or have increased requirements:

Pregnant women often need extra doses of some vitamins, especially folic acid (but *not* vitamin A).

Women whose periods are heavy may require iron (see page 18). *Elderly people* sometimes cut back on foods that supply vitamins, such as fresh vegetables and fruit, and may benefit from multivitamin and mineral supplements.

In heavy drinkers, alcohol depletes vitamin C and B vitamins.

Smokers use up vitamin C faster than nonsmokers.

Teenagers (as every mother knows) are either (a) compulsive consumers of junk food; (b) attempting to diet, or (c) turn vegetarian without compensating for the vitamins and minerals in meat. In a recent Department of Health survey, 90 per cent of adolescent girls turned out to be deficient in iron, 50 per cent in calcium (essential to prevent osteoporosis later in life), 60 per cent in riboflavin (needed to release energy) and 100 per cent in vitamin D (necessary to absorb calcium).

VITAMIN WHO'S WHO

The antioxidant vitamins

Antioxidants are hot news at the moment because of their newfound ability to seek out and de-activate 'free radicals'. These are molecules that are produced constantly in the body and exist for only a few seconds – but long enough to damage DNA, the genetic material in the cells, and trigger chain reactions in the arteries that could lead to heart attacks and other health problems. Chemicals, cigarette smoke, industrial pollution and radiation are also blamed for creating free radicals.

Vitamin A: found in liver, butter, cheese, margarine, eggs, carrots, tomatoes, apricots, oily fish, spinach and broccoli. Promotes good vision; needed to maintain healthy skin and mucous membranes; may protect against some cancers in the form of its precursor, **beta carotene**, which is an antioxidant that makes vitamin E more effective. Overdosing on vitamin A could cause birth defects in unborn children, harms the liver and causes blurred vision and headaches.

Vitamin C: found in oranges and other citrus fruits, blackcurrants, strawberries, kiwi fruit, tomatoes, spinach and other dark green vegetables, mango, and papaya. Promotes healthy gums and teeth; aids iron absorption and wound healing; may protect against some cancers as an antioxidant.

Vitamin E: found in nuts, vegetable oils, whole grains, olives, asparagus, spinach, tuna in oil, eggs, avocado, muesli, blackberries, wholemeal bread, brown rice, and salmon. Protects body tissues by preventing polyunsaturates being oxidised and forming free radicals. Important in the formation of red blood cells. A recent study at Harvard Medical School showed that vitamin E in supplement form is a powerful protector against heart disease.

B vitamins – the energy helpers

You need these to keep your nervous system in trim and to release energy from food during digestion. Likely sources are starchy foods, whole grains, meat and milk, and – welcome news for desperate mums and happy snackers – fortified breakfast cereals.

Vitamin B1 (Thiamine): found in whole grains, brown rice, nuts, bulghur wheat, wholemeal pasta and bread, dried beans, lean meats (especially pork), fish, and yeast extract. Vitamin B1 is needed to turn food into energy, the amount required depending on the amount of food eaten. Big appetites need more thiamine.

Vitamin B2 (Riboflavin): found in nuts, dairy products, liver, yeast extract, eggs, green leafy vegetables, lentils, and lean meat. Helps turn food into energy. Active people need more than couch potatoes.

Vitamin B3 (Niacin): found in nuts, dairy products, liver, oily fish, chicken, turkey, wholemeal bread, brown rice, and yeast extract. Vitamin B3 is involved in the synthesis of DNA, and the release of energy from food.

Vitamin B6: found in whole grains, dried beans, eggs, nuts, oats, fish, liver, brown rice, bananas, green leafy vegetables, wholemeal bread, and yeast extract. Vitamin B6 is involved in brain functioning and the formation of red blood cells. Again, the amount you need depends on how much protein you eat. Nutritionists deny widespread claims that pregnant and breastfeeding women and those on oral contraceptives need extra supplements.

Vitamin B12: found in liver, kidney, beef, eggs, milk, cheese, yoghurt, shellfish, sardines in oil, red meat, white and oily fish, and eggs. Vitamin B12 helps protect the nerves and prevent pernicious anaemia (see page 19). A few people who can't absorb vitamin B12 in the stomach receive it through injection, which started a notion that vitamin B12 'liver shots' could buck up the tired and weary and give added vigour. Forget it. Nutritional scientists are adamant that extra B12 won't alleviate ordinary fatigue or make anyone feel 'up to scratch'.

Vitamin D: found in milk, oily fish – mackerel, herring, kipper, tinned salmon, sardines, tuna and pilchard, brown rice, eggs, butter and margarine. Our skin makes vitamin D in response to natural sunlight. It's not really a vitamin but a hormone necessary for the absorption of calcium, needed for bones and teeth. Children who don't get enough vitamin D (now rare in Western societies) can develop rickets.

FOLATES

This is the name given to a group of substances made from folic acid, which is found in liver, kidney, wheat bran, leafy green vegetables, beans, grains, nuts, wholemeal bread, citrus fruit, eggs, brown rice, fresh and dried fruit and fortified breakfast cereals. Folates are important in the synthesis of DNA, and supplements are recommended for pregnant women.

THE MIGHTY MINERALS

Although our bodies contain only tiny amounts of most minerals, we can't survive without them. Without the 0.0004 per cent of us that is iodine, for instance, our thyroid gland could pack up. Originally part of the earth's crust, minerals are picked up from the soil, groundwater and sea by plants and animals and find their way into our food.

Quite how they work, or how much of each mineral is needed is still a subject for hot debate. That doesn't mean you should swallow bucketfuls in the hope of enhancing performance. Our bodies are so finely tuned and the interactions between one nutrient and another so complex that overdosing on one thing can throw others off balance. Too much extra calcium, for example, seems to interfere with the absorption of iron and other minerals.

But because minerals are uncharted territory, someone is always claiming magical properties for one or another. Chromium to cure hypoglycaemia! Phosphorus to reduce stress! Manganese to help fatigue! The fact is that nobody really knows.

Eating the varied and sensible diet suggested above should provide you with all you need. Take **manganese**, which is necessary for bone growth and cell function: it accounts for less than 0.005 per cent of our body and we absorb it fairly effortlessly from nuts, whole grains, vegetables, fruits, tea, instant coffee (!) and egg yolks.

Nevertheless there are some important minerals that it's easy to slip up on. Too much can be as bad as not enough, and many people overdose on **sodium**, which has been linked to hypertension, heart attacks and strokes, by wielding too heavy a hand with the salt cellar.

Calcium is important for strong bones, and women in particular need a calcium-rich diet so that their bones won't crumble with osteoporosis after menopause. Find it in full and low fat milk, cheese, yoghurt, spinach, tinned fish and eggs.

Iron (see page 18) is necessary to carry oxygen to the cells of the body. Not enough and you can become feeble with anaemia. Those at risk include: menstruating women, dieters (especially women), pregnant women, vegetarians, children and teenagers. Find it in liver, shellfish, dried fruits, dark green leafy vegetables, wholemeal bread, pulses and red meat. Lay off tea – tannin inhibits the absorption of iron. Vitamin C, on the other hand, gives it a helping hand.

Selenium is a mineral tripping off everyone's tongue these days. It works hand in hand with vitamin E to battle the dreaded free radicals. Find it in liver, kidney, white fish, tuna, shellfish, red meat, egg yolks, chicken, garlic, tomatoes, muesli, wholegrain cereals and wholemeal bread.

Zinc is essential for normal growth and sexual development. Not enough and puberty is delayed, wounds refuse to heal, and your sense of taste and smell go up the creek. It may have a role in fatigue – at least one British psychiatrist reports low levels of zinc and magnesium in people with depression who complain of feeling tired all the time. Find it in liver, lamb, beef, bacon, pork, oysters, eggs, turkey, breakfast cereals, cheese, and wholemeal bread.

Magnesium is known to help bone growth and the function of nerves and muscle. Find it in wheat bran, whole grains, raw leafy green vegetables, nuts (especially almonds and cashews), soy beans, bananas, apricots, spices.

Iodine is essential for the normal functioning of the thyroid gland and so may have a role in preventing fatigue. It has the agreeable bonus of keeping skin clear, nails strong and hair lustrous. Find it in iodised salt, seafood, seaweed food products, vegetables grown in iodine-rich areas and vegetable oil.

Two minerals commonly claimed to alleviate fatigue (though without convincing evidence as yet) are phosphorus and potassium. **Phosphorus** is important in energy metabolism. Find it in almost all foods, especially meats, poultry, fish, egg yolks, milk, dried peas and beans and nuts.

Potassium promotes a regular heartbeat, helps muscles contract, transfers nutrients to cells and controls water balance. Find it in oranges, bananas, dried fruits, peanut butter, dried peas and beans, coffee, tea, yoghurt, cocoa, and meat.

HOW SERIOUSLY SHOULD WE TAKE FOOD FADDISTS?

You only have to go into a chemist, let alone a health-food shop, to see just how popular – and how lucrative – is the food supplement business. Millions of pounds is invested in bottles and packets of multivitamins, phosphorus, chromium picolinate, evening primrose oil, algae, amino acids such as phenylalanine, herbal remedies such as ginseng and echinacea and heaven knows what else.

Feeling tired all the time? Try kelp tablets, say the health food producers. They're stiff with iodine, so they'll prevent your thyroid getting sluggish and keep the metabolism ticking along. Who knows? Or what about the amino acid L-glutamine? It's claimed that students taking it during exams think more clearly and remember more information.

Listening to the arguments for each is like tuning into the Tower of Babel, and if you followed all the sales pitches you'd be swallowing more pills and capsules than actual food. Few rigorous scientific studies (i.e., those not sponsored and promoted by supplement manufacturers) have turned up incontrovertible evidence for their claims. Even the glamorous evening primrose oil appeared in a recent trial to make little measurable difference to PMT symptoms – and yet thousands of women swear that it has calmed their mood swings and boosted their energy.

Maybe somebody ought to market the placebo effect. In many medication trials substantial numbers of people insist they feel better – even though they have been given a dummy rather than the active drug. In one trial of an anti-ulcer drug, 60 per cent of those on the placebo said their ulcers healed, compared with 70 per cent on the real thing. A demonstration, if ever one was needed, of the healing power of the mind.

If taking a daily vitamin and mineral tablet allows you some personal responsibility for your health, and you can afford to do so (food supplements don't come cheap) then who's to say that the mental and emotional benefits are not as great as any chemical ones?

'I take a vitamin A, C, E and selenium tablet daily, *and* an evening primrose oil capsule to supply gammalinolenic acid for cell growth,' says Prue, a health journalist. 'Okay, so I'm hedging my bets, hoping to offset any possible deficiencies. I live in a city, and because there's evidence that pollution from car exhausts and cigarette smoke can overwhelm the antioxidant defences in the lungs, I hope the vitamins will restore them. We don't have much control over our environment in general, so this is something I can *do*. And don't tell me that every apple has the same amount of nutrients, or that the lettuce wilting in the greengrocers' for five days has anything like the goodness of the one growing in my mother's garden.'

It's one thing to take a little garlic or vitamin C, but the meganutrient lobby pursues a more aggressive approach. They argue that we need massive doses of nutritional supplements to counter pollution, postpone ageing, increase energy levels and achieve ever higher peaks of health. No pussy-footing around here with a measly 100 mg of vitamin C; let's go for 5,000 or 10,000 mg. 5,000 iu of beta carotene? 25,000 iu is more like it. Be warned: mainstream nutritionists regard such high supplements as food faddery, dismissing them as rubbish and in some cases even dangerous.

Other dietary therapies need qualified supervision. Those who take **tissue salts** and **celloids**, which are special mineral supplements, swear by them, especially for cases of persistent fatigue, but you must consult a nutrition therapist and fill out a comprehensive symptom questionnaire before embarking on a course.

Naturopaths, who operate on the principle of helping the body to cure itself, will often recommend **supervised fasting** to clear the system of toxins accumulated by eating too much unhealthy food and living in stressful, polluted conditions. As you would have to be in solitary confinement on a Welsh hillside and devouring organic vegetables to avoid such horrors as petrol fumes and food additives, this probably applies to most of us.

Detoxification diets can be more demanding than you would imagine. I once spent several days with five others in a very beautiful Somerset house on a detoxification programme called Stop The World. We all arrived tired, stressed and knotted up in various ways and embarked on a diet of fresh fruit, raw vegetables, herbal teas and a truly disgusting cleansing drink called 'liverflush', allegedly made of olive oil, lemon juice, root ginger and garlic and intended to do exactly what its name suggests.

By the second day half of us had headaches, one person was vomiting, and another had back pain so severe she couldn't move. By the third day people were in tears, reliving past traumas. The organisers gave soothing aromatherapy massage, held and listened to sophisticated adults who were behaving like seven-year-olds. Astonishingly, by the fifth day, eyes were sparkling, skin was clear, and everyone went about saying 'my dear, I have never felt so wonderful, so free, so full of energy.'

CAN FOOD CHANGE YOUR MOOD?

Obvious examples of mood-changing foods are **alcohol** and **caffeine**.

A glass or two of wine a day, a single whisky or a pint of beer won't do any harm and, according to some studies, could do some good by reducing the risk of heart disease. In such moderation, **alcohol** relaxes tension, eases friendship and conversation, and makes the world less grey.

On the other hand, you don't *need* alcohol. Nutritionally, it's nothing but sugar, 'empty' calories, and toxins from which the body has to purge itself. Too much leaves you short of B vitamins, vitamin C and minerals. Because it's a diuretic, you'll pee more frequently and lose even more vitamins. It can mess up your sleep, block REM (rapid eye movement) dreaming necessary to help the brain deprogramme, intensify depression and impair the immune function. Instead of lifting your fatigue it will make it worse. Think of all that next time you're tempted to order another round.

Caffeine has a dubious reputation too. It's a stimulant drug, for a start – albeit one of the most popular and ancient. Western civilisation mops up caffeine by the gallon – in coffee, tea, cocoa, headache remedies, and soft drinks. An average coffee drinker can put away three cups a day without thinking twice, and aficionados dwell lovingly over that first freshly-brewed cup of the day. 'Damn fine coffee,' said Agent Cooper in *Twin Peaks*, and half the television audience rushed to put on the kettle.

This is what caffeine can do:

★ Step up your heartbeat and your metabolism.
★ Increase your stomach acid secretion and urine production.
★ Dilate some blood vessels and constrict others.
★ Fend off drowsiness and increase alertness.

In a recent study, a cup of coffee mid-morning was shown to improve concentration and motivation.

But it can also cause so-called coffee jitters – trembling, nervousness, chronic muscle tension, irritability, throbbing headaches, disorientation, sluggishness, depression and insomnia. Students who pour cup after cup into themselves to keep awake may find themselves revolving-eyed with fatigue, yet unable to relax.

Caffeine affects some people more than others, and those who drink it regularly seem to take most of these side effects in their stride. As with alcohol, moderation is the key. If you like a cup of coffee to keep you going mid-morning or tea for a lift in the afternoon, there's no reason why you shouldn't enjoy it. But if it keeps you awake at night, then it makes sense to avoid it after lunchtime. And remember that percolated or drip coffee contains twice as much caffeine as instant.

Some studies have hinted at links with heart disease and cancer, but none have been confirmed by further research. It's obviously sensible, though, to avoid coffee if you suffer heart arrhythmia.

Heavy coffee drinkers (six or more cups a day) could find that cutting it out too abruptly will give them withdrawal symptoms – headaches, lethargy, irritability, depression, nausea. Try cutting back gradually and switching to decaffeinated coffee.

Coffee for breakfast is fine, but not on its own. Fruit juice, cereals, wholemeal toast and yoghurt or milk is just what you need to launch you on the day. Teachers have observed that children who skip breakfast have a shorter concentration span.

Blood sugar levels need priming after twelve hours or so of fasting, and a combination of energy-releasing complex carbohydrate and protein is a better kickstart than the saturated fats in the traditional British fry-up of bacon, sausage, eggs, toasted white bread, butter and jam.

Too much fat in a meal dulls the brain. Who can help dozing off after the roast beef, Yorkshire pud and apple pie at Sunday lunch, when the generous helping of saturated fats makes red blood cells clump together so less oxygen reaches the brain? You feel h-e-a-v-y and s-l-e-e-p-y.

Energy levels dip in the body clock's post-lunch nadir anyway, so beat early afternoon fatigue by sticking to complex carbohydrates. Order spaghetti at lunch, rather than meat and chips and the cheeseboard.

Then in the evening, when you have supper before going to bed, let tryptophan in milk and bananas release serotonin, the brain's sleep-inducing hormone. Zzzzz.

EAT UP AND GO

Cabbage, full of selenium, is said to be good for anaemia, fatigue and stress. Eat it raw.

Sesame seeds are tiny storehouses of energy, rich in essential fatty acids and enzymes.

Sunflower seeds are packed with B vitamins such as thiamine, protein, iron and vitamin E.

Basil has a mild calming action that clears the head. Chop it in salads and add to pesto sauce, a perfect partner for high carbohydrate pasta.

Liver is stuffed with goodness: iron, zinc, vitamin A and all the vitamin B complex.

Rosemary is said to stimulate the adrenal cortex and step up the memory. Use it in cooking.

Guarana combats fatigue and aids concentration, according to South American Indians. It contains guaranine, a chemical similar to caffeine, but without the same side effects.

Guarana, Royal Jelly and Ginseng in Honey from Boots fights fatigue. Sip a 10ml. phial thirty minutes before strenuous mental or physical activity for an extra boost.

Reference

Eat for Life by Janette Marshall and Anne Heughan (Arrow)

CHAPTER 9

Get fit to fight fatigue

FIT FOR LIFE

Throwing yourself into physical exercise when you already feel exhausted seems madness. The last thing one would want to do. Surely *not* moving, lying down for a little rest, would be a more suitable occupation for a tired person?

Well, there's nothing wrong with little rests (I'm the first person to advise a restorative nap!) – in their place and at the right moment. But regular exercise, the aerobic kind that gets the lungs huffing, the heart racing, and oxygen rushing around every cell of the body, does more to dispel depression and fight fatigue than hours slumped in front of the telly.

Not only does a pepped-up circulation energise the body systems, it carries away toxins and waste products. All that spare adrenalin hanging over from your argument with the accounts manager and your frustration at sitting in a traffic jam for an hour? Gone. Sweated out.

So many modern occupations involve sitting down that people frequently have to be re-introduced to the benefits of physical activity. Our mothers and grandmothers walked to the shops, our grandfathers walked to work, and country children thought nothing of walking three miles to school. Nowadays a phalanx of cars is waiting for youngsters when classes finish, and there's a moan if anyone suggests a ten-minute stroll to the video shop.

And yet the physiological advantages of regular exercise are obvious. Excess weight vanishes, muscles are tauter, the heart beats better, lungs take in more air. Because your heart is pumping more blood per beat, the heart rate will drop lower when at rest. High blood pressure falls and the risk of heart disease is reduced. The levels of 'good' (HDL) cholesterol that protects against heart attack are raised. And it's cumulative: the more you exercise, the more your cells can produce and store energy. You'll hum like a little powerhouse.

Now there's proof that you'll feel better *psychologically* too – something committed exercisers usually take for granted, puffing back from a workout or a jog with that jolly-hockey-sticks glow. But it's more than a mere lifting of mood. American research shows exercise can treat mild depression as effectively as psychotherapy.

Stress levels are lower in fit people. In one study, inactive students were put on an aerobic programme of brisk walking or jogging for 35 to 40 minutes three times a week. After fourteen weeks they were given a series of unsolvable problems and told their results would be critical for their academic career (pity the poor students – they are put through hell in the interests of science). After the exam, those who exercised had lower blood pressure and lower levels of anxiety and muscle tension than non-exercisers.

In another study, when 2,500 sedentary people (i.e. couch potatoes whose idea of a workout is trundling a trolley round the supermarket) took up regular exercise, they reported significantly more energy and less tension than before.

It can affect your personality too. At Purdue University in the US, middle-aged sedentary people became emotionally more stable, self-sufficient, imaginative and confident after four months' regular exercise.

Mind you, it stands to reason that you'll feel better about yourself if you look in the mirror and see a trimmer waist and firmer muscles. Not to mention a sense of achievement. If you can do this, you can do anything. The positive knock-on effect of feeling more capable and in control includes an ability to concentrate and forge on even when tired.

Exercise stimulates the brain to release pain-killing hormones called endorphins. Runners talk of reaching a peak beyond fatigue and pain where they achieve a 'high', an addictive sense of well-being.

With all these amazing benefits, why aren't more of us out there thrashing about, working off stress hormones and buzzing with brain chemicals? An estimated 80 per cent of the population is unfit. People take up exercise regimes and drop them again. The number of unused exercise bicycles gathering dust in British homes doesn't bear thinking about.

The unpalatable truth is that exercise (a) is often boring, and (b) it can take ages – a minimum of eight to twelve weeks – for any benefits to be noticeable.

Tamsin is a strong natural swimmer with a graceful style who excelled at long-distance events. When she left school, however, she gave up the sport. If she goes swimming now it's to lark about, never to do laps. 'Serious training is unbelievably dull,' she says. 'You have to do at least thirty or forty laps of an Olympic pool to keep in top shape, and it's numbing. Up and down, up and down. I couldn't stand any more.'

Those driven by a competitive spirit will keep it up, but what about the rest of us? We need a motivation other than the thrill of excelling. The image of the hyperathlete who works out daily, pumping away at exercise machines and treadmills, is daunting. Does it have to be quite so . . . rigorous?

The answer is no. Researchers at the University of Massachusetts and Harvard Medical Schools have found that relatively gentle exercise, combined with relaxation techniques, produces very positive results remarkably quickly.

Using the inevitable sedentary people – not hard to find – they sent some off to walk 'moderately' quickly for forty minutes three times a week while listening to relaxation tapes, and some to 'mindful' exercise classes that combined yoga and t'ai chi movements with music and imagery. Both programmes improved fitness and reduced anxiety and enhanced mood ten weeks earlier than those on a walking only regime. Engaging mind and body together packs a double whammy.

'It's tapping into positive thinking,' says Lisbeth Giampaolo, of the Espree Health Club, London, where similar programmes have been introduced. 'You can repeat your favourite story, a prayer, count breaths, say a mantra, or make positive affirmations – "I can do anything." Instead of pedalling on an exercise bike and thinking how horrible your job or your relationship is, you engage your mind in a positive way.'

Do I have to spend hours in the gym?

Not unless you want to. Aim for 15–60 minutes aerobic exercise a day, three to five days a week. Under three days, and you won't see any benefits; more than five is keen, but won't make a substantial difference in fitness.

If aerobic exercise is to do any good, your heart rate should reach what is called the training rate, between 70 and 90 per cent of the maximum. To find the right rate for you, subtract your age from 220 – the maximum heart rate (MHR) – and multiply that number by 0.6 and 0.8. This will give the lower and upper limits of your target heart rate during exercise.

Build the exercise into your daily schedule rather than getting up earlier in the morning (TATT sufferers cling to every last second in bed) or tagging it on after work, when you'll either be held up in a late-running meeting or so exhausted the last thing you'll want is to flog around a gym or pool.

Know thyself: don't be swayed by hardy souls who boast of swimming thirty lengths before breakfast. I once wasted £300 joining a health club near the office, because I thought I would get in at 8 a.m. for a workout. Alas, the spirit was willing, but the early morning flesh . . . I made it three times in the whole twelve months of membership.

Better to park the car a mile or two from the station and walk. Climb the stairs at the office rather than take the lift. Or drag your exercise bike out of mothballs and watch TV or read the newspaper while pedalling. The number of calories you can work off in an hour while engaged in the most mundane activities is extraordinary: in a 130 pound woman, cleaning the house (222 calories) and food shopping (222) almost equals cycling (228 at 5.5m.p.h.).

Once you have a regime going, eight weeks without exercising can put you back to square one, so if time is tight, don't drop it altogether. Keep up an abridged form so that you don't lose all the benefits.

Remember:

★ Set sensible goals. If you're flabby and out of condition, it's better to aim for ten minutes three times a week to start with, rather than plunging in to 45 minutes four times a week.

★ Choose a convenient form of exercise. If it takes three changes on the train and a bus ride to reach a swimming pool, you'll soon get sick of the travelling and feel a failure. And a tired one at that.

★ Vary the exercise. Walk one day, cycle the next.

★ Choose the right footwear. There's no point attempting power walking in the fashion shoes you wear to work.

★ Stop and rest if you feel dizzy or uncomfortable. You shouldn't push yourself so hard that you can't (just) hold a conversation at the same time.

★ Spend five or ten minutes warming up before aerobic exercise, and another five or ten winding down.

★ Check with your doctor if you suffer from high blood pressure, dizziness, heart disorders, back pain, diabetes or arthritis, or if you are over 45 and plan a particularly strenuous regime.

HOW FIT ARE YOU?

You may not really want to know this, but . . .

Step up, one foot after another, onto the bottom step of an ordinary staircase, then step down, one foot after another. Keep this up twice every five seconds for three minutes. If you get dizzy or feel faint, *stop*. When finished, rest for 30 seconds and take your pulse.

You are unfit if after exercise:

you are a man of 20–29 and your pulse rate is 102
              30–39   102
              40–49   106
              over 50   106

you are a woman of 20–29 and your pulse rate is 112
              30–39   114
              40–49   114
              over 50   118

A very fit man of 30–39 has a pulse rate after exercise of 78, and a very fit woman the same age has one of 86.

WHICH FORM OF EXERCISE TO CHOOSE?

Tired, tense and stressed-out people with overloaded schedules could be asking for trouble if they plump for competitive sports. Better to opt for the kind of exercise where you can pace yourself, or that you can do in company – but not in competition – with others. Keep it simple, too. The last thing you want is exercise that is complicated, involving a lot of organisation, travel and/or equipment.

Andy is a lawyer who takes his passion to win at all costs beyond the courtroom. 'I was pretty wound up and on the edge, so I joined a tennis club to play for relaxation and exercise, but I found it very stressful. I'd get so uptight over beating the hell out of my opponent my heart would race when I went on court, and the night after I lost the tournament semi-finals I could hardly sleep.'

Now he cycles – alone. 'Though I find myself racing cars . . .'

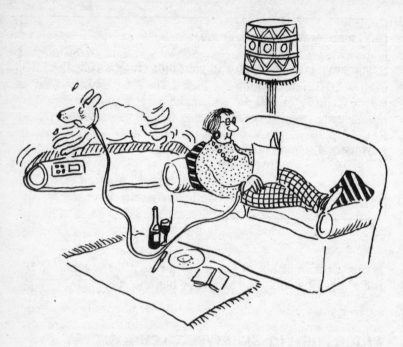

Aerobic movement classes

Look for low-impact aerobics. You'll get the same health benefits without jarring your body to bits.

Make sure the class suits you. Is it the right level? If you're out of condition, an advanced class will have you on your knees – or even in hospital. The shock of sudden exercise, especially if you're over 45 and not renowned for your activity, could be downright dangerous.

The teacher should begin with a warm-up and finish with a cooling down, sandwiched around twenty minutes of exercise that gets your heartbeat to the training rate. Beware instructors who swan about preening at their own performance. Notice whether he or she reminds people to check their pulse rates and actually watches the exercisers, instructing them when necessary and letting them work at their own speed.

Cycling
One of the simplest and most agreeable for someone who's tired and easily daunted by large classes and fancy equipment. Begin on a paved roadway that's fairly level – save the hills until your stamina builds up. Pick a 10–12 speed bike with a sturdy, lightweight frame and make sure it fits you, or your muscles will ache. A gentle cycling holiday (somewhere flat – France, perhaps?) has a certain charm as a way of easing yourself in.

Dancing
Have fun and make friends while exercising. Fans of Strictly Ballroom please note: you can burn off 250–300 calories per hour doing the rumba, the tango and the foxtrot.

Running and jogging
This is the aerobic sport par excellence. There's a kind of lonely joy in pounding along that takes you out of yourself. Begin by walking more and more briskly until you're running and can keep it up for half an hour. For goodness sake invest in proper shoes: they should bend at the ball where the foot does.

Skiing
Cross-country is best of all to get muscles and circulation hammering away, but difficult to organise if you live anywhere south of Leeds. Downhill won't work the heart and lungs quite so well, but you can still burn 420 calories an hour. Expensive to keep up unless you live on a Swiss mountain, but certainly one way of enjoying a healthy holiday.

Swimming
People swear by it as the ideal aerobic exercise. Heart, lungs and muscles all get a working out. Do the forward crawl for best effect, starting with four laps of 25 yards each with a rest between each lap, and gradually adding laps and decreasing the rests until you can swim continuously for 30–40 minutes. If it's boring, try some of the relaxation techniques described

above to occupy your mind. And buy a decent pair of goggles that fit if chlorine irritates your eyes and you can't see where you're going.

Tennis and badminton
If you're serious about aerobic exercise, you should play only singles and vigorously at that – leaping after balls and rushing about the court. Choose an opponent with a similar level of skill, so that you'll get some decent rallies.

Walking
Simple, safe and cheap – what more can you ask? You can do it anywhere: in city streets, suburban parks, country lanes, moors and mountains; on your own, with a companion, or a crowd.

Brisk walking – in which you walk fast, four and a half miles per hour, and pump your arms up and down – can provide nearly the same aerobic benefits as running. Swing your arms, using handweights – or substitute a briefcase or shopping bag, though take care to avoid swiping hapless passersby.

If you're inactive but healthy, begin by walking a mile at three miles per hour five times a week, and gradually increase to three miles at four miles per hour. Make sure your shoes have a cushioning heel and toe, especially on city pavements.

At weekends, get out for a country hike and tackle a few hills. Remember to dress for outdoor exercise, with layers of loose, thin garments that can be shed as you start to sweat, and are light enough to knot around your shoulders or waist. And take a water bottle – you'll need to replace the fluids lost through perspiration.

What do I think? This is personal witness time: halfway through writing this chapter I was so tired I wanted to shut my eyes and let it all float away. Instead – deeming it wise in the circumstances to take my own advice – I forced myself on a 25-minute fast walk through the park. The sun shone and children played on the grass. I came back nicely puffed, had a long drink of water, and – yes, dear reader – sat down again to the word processor with a clear head and renewed vigour.

MIND AND BODY EXERCISE

Rushing about and getting breathless isn't the only form of exercise that will keep you physically fit. Others emphasise the partnership of the mind with the body, concentrating on stre-e-e-tching muscles on the wave of the breath.

Yoga

Simple yoga breathing and stretching exercises (pranayama) boost mental and physical energy better than almost anything. Psychologists at Oxford University recently found that 30 minutes of yoga was more effective than relaxation or visualisation (imagining your energy and ways to increase it).

Hardly an adult education centre in the country is without its yoga class, working their way through the Cobra, the Triangle and the Half Shoulder Stand (the latter especially recommended for tiredness). You can almost touch the atmosphere of concentration, as poses are stretched into, held, and breathed with.

'I love it,' says Jordan, a 34-year-old actor. 'There's not many forms of exercise that strengthen your muscles and keep your mind so calm and lucid. Afterwards I feel very resilient and somehow secure.'

The exotically-named poses (Tadasana – the mountain, Vrksasana – the tree) are designed to encourage flexibility, good posture, muscle co-ordination and controlled breathing, which in turn increase blood circulation, bring a feeling of relaxation and well-being and release the mind from tension. Yoga teachers have a way of looking incredibly supple and serene, so they must be on to a good thing.

On the whole, Britons are more interested in yoga as a method of keeping fit, so the physically-oriented forms such as hatha and Iyengar are most popular. Other yoga systems that emphasise the intellect and the morals are still largely unknown in this country.

Yoga can be learnt from books but you're well advised to attend a class to make sure you're doing it right before practising at home.

References

The British Wheel of Yoga,
   1 Hamilton Place,
   Boston Road,
   Sleaford,
   Lincolnshire NG34 7ES
   (tel. 0529 306851)

Yoga for Health Foundation,
   Ickwell Bury,
   Biggleswade,
   Bedfordshire SG18 9EF
   (tel. 0767 627271)

T'ai-chi Ch'uan (T'ai Chi)
This ancient Chinese technique has been called 'meditation in motion' and that is exactly what it looks like: slow, flowing, deliberate movements that demand the mind's full attention, an extraordinary combination of relaxation and control. In this way *Qi* (life energy) is balanced and moves smoothly through the body to combat stress and disease and maintain physical and mental harmony.

People in frantic high-pressure jobs have found T'ai Chi an alternative to tranquillisers, and the sight of workers by the roadside in China, intent on these steady, graceful movements is remarkably soothing. To stand in the open air and perform steps with names like 'the stork cools its wings' and 'strumming the lute' must be supremely pleasing.

T'ai Chi must be learnt – it can't really be picked up in books.

Information about classes and teachers is available from The School of T'ai Chi Ch'uan.

Reference

The School of T'ai Chi Ch'uan,
   5 Tavistock Place,
   London WC1H 9SS

BREATHING

This is as good a place as any to think about breathing, and reflect on the astonishing fact that vast numbers of people breathe in quite the wrong way.

What? I hear you protest. But breathing is what we do from the moment we're born. Breathing is what keeps us alive.

All true. But there are two main types of breathing. Costal breathing (costal meaning the ribs) is the kind of shallow chest breathing that we do when exercising vigorously or feeling stressed and panicky.

People who do it too quickly and too often (as in panic attacks) hyperventilate – they become light-headed and lose consciousness because the blood tension of carbon dioxide is lowered (breathing into a paper bag, the classic remedy, increases the intake of CO_2). Needless to say, it is a very tiring way of staying alive, especially when you are breathing like this most of the time.

Abdominal or diaphragmatic breathing uses the diaphragm, the sheet of muscle between the chest cavity and the abdomen. Breathe in and the diaphragm pushes downwards, the tummy rises, and the lungs expand, taking in a good whack of oxygen. Breathe out, the diaphragm relaxes, the abdomen sinks and the lungs expel air containing carbon dioxide. This kind of breathing pumps energising oxygen into all the body and brain tissues, and is one of the best ways possible to reduce stress and overcome fatigue.

Check that you are breathing from the diaphragm by lying on your back and putting one hand on your chest and the other on your abdomen. Notice which hand is moving when you breathe in and out. If it's the hand on your chest, then you're breathing the wrong way. Concentrate on pulling in your tummy muscles, pushing them in if necessary with your hand, to train yourself to breathe deeply from the diaphragm.

Energy booster

Picture your breath carrying a boost of dynamic energy to all the tired and sluggish parts of your body.

Stand up, close your eyes and take a deep breath, feeling your tummy expand. Slowly raise your arms out from your sides and above your head. Stretch as you breathe out and bring down your arms.

Breathe in, raise your arms again and imagine your breath as a wave of energy sweeping through your body, waking up every cell and filling it with vigour.

Breathe out and bring your arms down. Repeat this three times.

Pay attention to any area that feels tense, such as your shoulders. When you breathe in, picture your breath carrying the life energy to that area, warming it and revitalising it.

Repeat this with any other tense areas until all are energised by the power of your breath.

On the in-breath, stretch your palms to the ceiling and then slowly bring your arms back to your side. Feel how refreshed and light your body is.

One-breath fix

If you're stuck in a traffic jam or behind your desk and feeling jaded, give yourself an energy fix. Take a deep breath and imagine the energy sweeping through you, enlivening every muscle and nerve-ending from the top of your head to your fingertips and toes. Breathe out and relax.

CHAPTER 10

Take a good look at yourself

SELF-KNOWLEDGE

Remember Alison? Back in Chapter 6? Alison, the head of music at a further education college, who crumpled under a burden of fatigue and stress? Under doctor's orders to rest at home for three weeks, she was forced to take stock of her life. Her mind and body had issued an ultimatum: something had to give.

'At first, when I stopped feeling quite so tired, I was tempted to ignore it all. Then the thought of going back into the office made me panicky again. And, instead of being stuck in a meeting, I found I enjoyed being around the house in the early evening when the children came in and we could natter in a comfortable way. As I stopped nagging and shouting at them, making them the scapegoats of my own misery and frustration, my son and I began talking again, and Trish's school work picked up.'

She and Jim, her husband, made time for a long weekend away on their own, something they had not done for years. 'It's funny how, at home where everything has become routine, you end up communicating in grunts, taking things for granted. Jim was as familiar to me as the wallpaper in the sitting room and seemed to need as little conversation. But in a different setting, we looked at each other as people again. We talked about what was happening in our lives, how we felt about each other and the children and our jobs. I was able to *listen* when Jim told me about his fears about redundancy, instead of shoving it under the carpet. We found ourselves giggling and joking in a way we'd forgotten, and after dinner, all talked out and mellow with wine, we made love as we hadn't done for years. It was *all right*.

'I discovered that Jim and I were okay, our relationship wasn't as hollow and dead as I'd feared – though God knows if we would have been able to retrieve it if things had gone on the way they were going.'

In her time at home, Alison thought very carefully about what she really valued in her life, and how it could be accommodated. One thing was clear: she could not allow herself to wind up in such a state again, but how to avoid it? Her gut reaction was to hand in her notice, but in the current economic climate Jim's job with a publishing company was insecure and there were bills to be paid. She consulted the children, Rory and Trish: What did her job mean for them? What would they like to see changed?

Surprisingly – to Alison, at any rate – the response of both children was very mature. They understood the financial situation and the need for Alison to work. If only she could be more available for them. They, too, liked having her home at five thirty, in time for tea, instead of eight. Not necessarily *every* night, they conceded – they accepted there were occasions a couple of times a week when she had to be late.

'What do I need to change if I am going to continue in this job? And what can I do if I don't?' Alison asked herself. A change of college principal would be wonderful, but that *was* something beyond her power. She knew she didn't have the temperament or the will to engage in internal politicking.

She narrowed her requirements down to four key points:

1. Her hours must be more flexible to allow her to leave earlier.
2. She needed training and help with her administrative skills. She was aware, for example, that she could delegate more if only she knew how.
3. She had to make space for her own musical expression. 'When I don't play, my life juices dry up,' she acknowledges.

4. She needed more practical help in the house if she was to have any emotional energy left over for Jim and the children.

So important was it that these criteria be met, she decided, that if they were not, she would go back to teaching music, privately if necessary, for a living. The salary would be less, but they would get by – and at least Jim still had his job, however tenuously.

'In a curious way, making that "worst possible scenario" decision gave me strength,' she says. She put her case to the principal who, recognising the determination behind her reasonable manner, agreed that she would be free to leave college at 5 p.m. at least three days a week. He also agreed to her request for management training.

It hasn't always been easy, but Alison has been firm about keeping to her new timetable. 'It's meant that I've had to be ruthless about not being available for last-minute late meetings, and that some days I go in early to keep up with work, but by and large, it's okay. The principal leaves me alone more – I think, in a funny way, I earned his respect. Anyway, he has enough problems these days with other staff members.'

She has joined a small group of local musicians, who play once a week for pleasure, and occasionally in public. She and Jim make a point of spending time together out of the house once a week; the children are more willing and Jim is readier to help out with the cooking and washing up. 'I still do the lion's share of organising,' says Alison, 'but he's come a long way for a man of his generation, brought up to think the kitchen is a woman's place.'

Executives and dealers on their knees with exhaustion are nothing new for Jane McWhirter, a McTimoney chiropractor and director of All Hallows House, a centre for complementary medicine in the City of London. 'The ethos is one of hype and buzz buzz buzz,' she says. 'They have to keep themselves revved up because they're dealing with three phones and screens and colleagues simultaneously. They need rest, but their bodies are not in a state to use it, and these people get so low, so out of touch and wound up, that they don't benefit from the sleep they do get in the ordinary way.'

The first questions she asks are about their way of life. 'Where they're at. What their motivation is. What they want to do with their life. Often they're caught up in situations that are eating their energy away. They're not getting enough support from their partners, they're in the wrong job, or they feel they have to overwork to be acknowledged. We ask them to stop and make the time and space for reassessment.'

When you're on that kind of treadmill it can seem a mad indulgence to waste time in self-contemplation. 'If I stopped and thought about what I'm doing I mightn't like it,' said a young woman in property investment. Well, quite. But how far can you go in a job that, deep down, is not something you admire? Or that devours all your psyche, so that you have no inner spaces in which to withdraw for renewal? What will that do for your self-esteem? Or your powers of recuperation?

Too far down that path, and the crash – or the burnout – when it comes can be catastrophic. Everything's up in the air. Marriages founder, careers are abandoned. Jane knows of cases where people, pushed to the limits of their endurance, have rebelled and thrown in high salary jobs. 'And yet, if they'd been able to balance their lives better before exhausting themselves, they might have maintained their jobs quite happily for years to come.' Sometimes only a minor change – leaving work an hour earlier, keeping Sundays free for relaxation – can put circumstances into a low enough gear to be manageable.

But switching tracks really might be the best solution. For one reason or another – your parents wanted it, your best friend was doing it – we can drift into a career for which we were never cut out. Nothing is more debilitating than being in the wrong job.

JOB SATISFACTION

For six endless months I once worked for a small public relations company. The difference between journalism and public relations may not appear great (and for many it's an effortless transfer from one to the other), but in one of those great learning curves of life, I discovered that promoting products – especially ones that in normal circumstances I would avoid like the plague – is not something at which I am very good. In fact I was hopeless.

Among our accounts there was a restaurant chain so down-market that steak and chips were cordon bleu fare, and a maternity wear manufacturer (this was pre-babies for me) in whose garments I wouldn't have been seen dead, even if I was expecting triplets. I struggled to muster enthusiasm, but it was a miserable charade. Every morning I woke up dreading going into work; I was depressed and always tired and I felt a failure. Why couldn't I, too, feign boundless excitement over chicken-in-a-basket and Black Forest Gateau, served amid an indigestible decor of Mock Tudor and – for some reason a nautical theme being part of the chain's image – Walt Disney Pirate Ship?

And then one happy day I was offered a job on a newspaper again, and suddenly the sun shone and I felt so alive I wanted to sing.

Job satisfaction (and this includes unpaid work in the home or the voluntary sector) is the elusive factor that is all-important. Why can some people handle what appear to be horrendously stressful careers with aplomb? Susie is a fashion designer who flies to Europe or Hong Kong at least once a week as well as organising a home and three children, and she thrives on it. She's in a job she adores and does well, and so if she has jet lag for a day or two, or is getting by on four hours' sleep a night because her new range is coming out, then it's manageable. A couple of nights' good rest and she's restored to full wattage.

Without job satisfaction, however, not only will your work

suffer because your heart (literally) isn't in it, but so will your health. More people keel over with a heart attack at 9 a.m. on Monday mornings (the 'Black Monday' syndrome) than any other time of the week, and they invariably turn out to be chronically unhappy in their job.

Psychologist Suzanne Kobasa in the US found that company managers under the same amount of stress fell into two groups: one half complained of endless health problems, including persistent fatigue, and the other half did not. The healthy individuals were the kind who would describe a cup as half full, rather than half empty. They lived according to what she called the Three Cs. Stress they saw as a *Challenge*, something natural and inevitable; they believed themselves to be in *Control* of their workload; and they had a *Commitment*, not only to their job, but to their families and to life in general.

How does one achieve this constructive state of mind? Begin with yourself and what, and where, you are now.

GET TO KNOW YOURSELF

Escape for a few days if you can. Being outside your normal environment can cast a different light on what had seemed an absolutely impossible situation.

For some, a retreat house can provide peace and space for evaluation. Holiness is not a requisite – although feeling comfortable in a spiritual atmosphere helps. There are Buddhist and New Age retreats as well as Christian that will welcome you.

Failing this, take a few hours off to be by yourself. Mooch around a park. Sit by the river. And take a notebook and pencil. This is an exercise in self-knowledge. The more acquainted you become with yourself, the easier it will be to control how you feel and behave. You'll be wasting less energy on dead-end areas and have more to tap for the things that really count.

Some of the exercises below will seem a bit daft if you're not in the habit of being introspective, but it's astonishing how we can bump along from one day to the next without seriously mulling over who we are, or what we can do, or even what we actually believe in.

How long will this state of affairs last?
Is this situation likely to go on forever – or the foreseeable future, at least? A purely practical question. Many exhausting projects are short term: one day soon I'll finish this book, and I can go to bed early and lie in the garden in the sun and read ten rubbishy novels all in a row.

Or take mothers with young children. Right now you may be drained from lack of sleep and endless claims on your time – privacy is something for which you retreat to the bathroom and lock the door – but *children do grow*. The demands on your energies will be different – teenagers have a way of wanting to talk about the Meaning Of Life or Do You Think I'm Too Young For Sex at eleven o'clock at night – but at least you'll eventually be free of that insistent physical fatigue.

What's happening in your life right now?
Draw a pie chart (this is something development counsellors love getting people to do in workshops, but it's still a thought-provoking exercise). Divide the slices of the pie according to how much time you spend at work and getting to work, how much time with your partner, your family, with friends, in community work (and this could mean helping out with the church fete or selling raffle tickets for Save The Children) and how much time for you, yourself – painting, reading, evening classes, whatever.

Now draw another pie chart with the slices the size you would like them to be. Think about the differences. What could you do to make the first chart match the second?

Where do I want to be in five years' time?
Don't worry about how far-fetched it might appear. What's wrong with famous best-selling novelist? Or head of an interna-

tional fashion house? Or owner of a pizza restaurant, for that matter? What could you do to achieve it? (Buying a word processor might be a start, or taking a course in business management.) What changes could you make – in your job, your qualifications, your relationships, your leisure time?

What are my good qualities?

What do I do well? Women are particularly abysmal at this. We've been so conditioned that it's improper for little girls to boast and be pushy, that we hesitate to allow ourselves any assets at all. Go on, swallow your embarrassment. 'I've got good legs' will do for a start. 'I'm a good organiser' might be another if you've just run the school jumble sale. If you can't think of anything nice off your own bat, remember compliments that you've been paid. Put the list beside your mirror or somewhere you'll see it regularly (inside your wardrobe door if you feel it looks a bit odd for public consumption) and add to it as new plusses occur.

What are my weaknesses?

Psychotherapist Gael Lindenfield recommends making a list of your failings, and then finding a positive side to each. 'A worrier' becomes 'careful thinker'. Very creative. Compile another list of your strengths, maybe borrowing from your positive 'failings'.

What are my values?

How we measure other people and events and the decisions we take about how we spend our time and money, are based on a set of beliefs that many of us have only half thought about. Some of these will be part of the baggage we grew up with ('it's wrong to steal') and some we have hammered out for ourselves ('the world should be free of pollution').

If our way of life contradicts any of them, then we're uneasy and unhappy and our energy dribbles away. If we feel buoyant and energised, on the other hand, then what we're doing fits comfortably with our values. Taking the kids on a picnic, for instance, will give you a buzz if you value being with your children. (Feeling energised doesn't necessarily mean bounding around sparking in all directions. Sitting listening to music you enjoy gives a pleasure and peace of mind that is full of restorative energy.)

Make four lists of the things you value – at work, in relationships, the world and yourself. This is your private list, for your eyes only, so don't con yourself by putting down noble ideas because you think they look good. 'Having a nice house' is as genuine a value as 'world peace'.

Then check to see where your values fit each other – and where they conflict. Your work list, for example, might include 'making money' or 'travel'. But how will these fit in with 'having a family', 'time to garden', or 'spiritual development'?

Now – this is an exercise Liz Willis puts to good effect in her development programme 'Springboard' – rank your values in terms of 'I *must* have', 'I would like to have', 'It would be nice to have.' Tick the ones that are being met and underline the ones that aren't. Any un-met values in the 'I *must* have' section will give you clues to your goals for the future.

What do I enjoy?
Psychologist Anne Dickson recommends this exercise in her book, *A Woman In Your Own Right – Assertiveness and You.* On a large sheet of paper write, on the left-hand side, twenty pleasures: simple – and perhaps not so simple – things that you enjoy. Walking in sand, the smell of wet grass after rain, the soft skin of a baby, your partner's voice after an absence, the anticipation of the theatre, the liberation of driving out of the city.

Then divide the rest of the page into three columns. In the first column, beside each pleasure, put a T for Together, or A for Alone, or T/A for both. In the second column, put a large £ if the pleasure is expensive, and a small £ if it's not. In the final column, write down how long since you have enjoyed it. Then consider what this tells you about yourself and your approach to pleasure. Do you have more pleasure by yourself, or with someone else? If there's something you haven't enjoyed for a long time, then why? Are there opportunities for pleasure around you every day? Is it hard for you to find pleasure?

Do I know my own body?
We are all – thank God – different. Some of us are blessed with physical stamina, and others with mental endurance. Of course we should eat well and exercise for optimum strength and fitness, but there will be a point at which we attain our peak – and that peak may not be as high as someone else's.

I've learnt to recognise certain signals, for instance, that mean I'm going into fatigue overload – eyelids twitch, I stammer, and I develop irrational obsessions. It's time to slow down and take steps to lighten the load. Esther Rantzen says that in her case exhaustion triggers a form of dyslexia; words break up on the page she's reading.

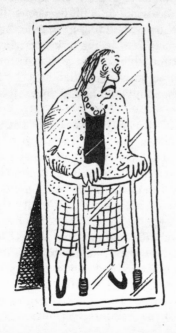
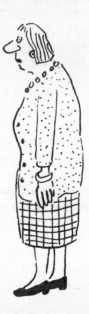

Watch your energy highs and lows. 'Owls' are slow to wake in the morning and come alive in the evening. 'Larks' rise with the sun and are ready to fold their wings once the supper plates are washed up.

A relationship between an Owl and a Lark needs a lot of understanding: when one is raving to go, the other wants to drop. But fatigue can be a real issue if circumstances force you out of your natural rhythm. Owl mothers crawl out of bed to get children to school; if the late nights add up they have an energy crisis. Try shifting your sleep schedule if you can, and identify new high energy periods for maximum output; late morning or afternoon perhaps.

WHAT NEXT?

This is the hard bit, where *you* have to make the applications to your own life, and maybe take some difficult decisions. It could mean cutting back on some areas, building in time for others.

If you're spending too much time in the office or travelling, can you restructure your timetable so that you work more at home? Or if you work at home, have you fallen into the trap of never closing the door on the study and giving yourself a night off?

Roger commuted four hours a day between Grantham in Lincolnshire and London – two hours on the train to Kings Cross, and two hours back. He left home at six every morning and in the evening – well, anything from 8 or 9 p.m. He only saw his children awake at weekends, and, being a man who derived not only much pleasure but a sense of identity from his family, this lack of contact began to nag at him. His longing to be at home with his wife and kids in the evenings, rather than swaying about on a commuter train, began to leak into his work. He grew resentful and impatient, he lost the ambition and the effervescent energy that had led him to attempt the daily journey in the first place, his back ached, his head ached and he complained of feeling tired all the time.

He reasoned he had two alternatives. (Three, if you count continuing with a schedule that was obviously fraying him apart at the seams.) The family could move closer to London, away from his and his wife's parents, and into a smaller house. Or he could change his job for one closer to home.

As so often happens when things reach a head and you start looking for ways out, just as he and his wife reluctantly put their house on the market, he was offered a job in Nottingham, just over half an hour's drive away. With one bound he was free.

It was not without sacrifice, however. Roger enjoyed the status of his big London company, and the Nottingham firm was smaller, although growing fast. But the compensations of spending time with the children and becoming involved in local activities – he became a school governor, which satisfied his craving for influence – were overwhelmingly more rewarding.

Ask yourself

Am I spending too much time travelling? (Don't assume all commuting is tiring. One survey revealed that people with long inter-city commutes found them less fatiguing because they could sit down and read, than those sandwiched for an hour in crowded suburban trains.)

Would I like to spend more time with the family?

When did my partner and I last have a conversation where we talked about our dreams and emotions?

Am I spending too much time at work in tasks I don't enjoy?

Do I have leisure interests that take me out of my work mode?

When did I last read a book for relaxation/go to the theatre/ movies/concert?

When did I last play tennis/swim/go for a hike in the country?

When did I last have a good laugh?

References

Springboard – Women's Development Workbook by Liz Willis and Jenny Daisley (Hawthorn Press)

Super Confidence by Gael Lindenfield (Thorsons)
The Vision annual programme of
The National Retreat Association,
  Liddon House,
  24 South Audley Street,
  London W1Y 5DL
  (tel. 071-493 3534)

CHAPTER 11

Getting your act together

ASSERTIVENESS TRAINING *OR* CONFIDENCE BUILDING *OR* BETTER AND BETTER

You've found your dream . . . It could be climbing the Himalayas, opening a children's boutique, studying law, spending Sunday mornings in bed, reading one good book a month or cycling to work to avoid the traffic and keep fit. *Anything*. It's *your* dream. But it's a good dream, because when it came to you your heart lifted and you had a flash almost of recognition.

For a moment your energy levels surge: 'This is it. My life will change. I'm free of the trap.'

And then everything plummets because you think: 'I haven't the time to do that.' 'Who'll get the family their supper if I join an evening class?' 'I daren't ask if I can work at home one day a week; they'll never allow it.' 'What's the point of learning to paint? I'm no good at art.' 'We can't afford a bicycle for me when Sam needs new golf clubs.' And on, and on. The old blanket of fatigue descends again.

The worst self-saboteurs, unfortunately, are women. More dreams have foundered on guilt than you would believe possible – and nobody, but nobody, is more bound and strapped by guilt than the working mother. If you rate guilt from 1 to 10, then she's up there at 9$\frac{1}{2}$ just because she wanted a career.

Times *are* changing, and many young mothers take it for granted they'll be back at the desk after maternity leave, but there's also a private, individual guilt. Guilt because you're not there when your child falls over and cries, or takes her first step, or you can't make the school sports day and he's tipped to win a cup. Guilt because you're taking home M&S chicken Kiev *yet again*, and you haven't time to stand over the stove making nourishing lentil and vegetable soup. And like most intractable, gnawing emotions – grief and jealousy are others – persistent guilt is debilitating; draining not so much physical energy as that of the spirit and imagination.

There was a dreadful period, round about the early eighties, when we rushed about being Superwoman. This meant terminal exhaustion and chronic guilt because you hurtled home from the office (where you had been Ms Perfect Power Shoulders) to bath the children, feed them fish fingers, pop a soufflé in the oven for your husband, plan the weekend dinner party for ten, iron a basket of shirts, cut out curtains and later make wild passionate love as if you'd had nothing better to do all day.

Thank God that has passed. The first woman who confessed that dust grew quite nicely in her corners thank you deserves a medal. But then the concept of juggling took its place; working mum as conjuror. You were allowed an element of trickery – cutting a corner here, patching it there – as long as you didn't actually drop one of the umpteen balls you were keeping in the air.

But *self*-indulgence – apart from the odd game of tennis or a trip to the hairdresser's – well now, that was asking too much. If you were out of the house cut-and-thrusting all week, then the least one could do was Be There at the weekend, and not gallivanting off on some airy-fairy personal development course.

Besides, such busy-busyness is curiously addictive. Juggling becomes as competitive as being Superwoman: look at clever me – I'm doing this and this and this, and never a mistake. And concentrating so much on what's up in the air takes the mind off where one's feet are. Best not to even *think* what the feet are doing (until, of course, one falls over). If I settled down for a lazy afternoon with a good book my guilt-ridden conscience hammered at my shoulder. What about the overflowing washing basket? Tidying out the toy box? A whole afternoon to spare? I could be cooking the week's meals in advance. Even distance was no escape. Twelve thousand miles away I'd find myself waking in a cold sweat. Had they switched off the iron? Fed the cat?

But there's a difference between feeling guilty and being responsible, and the trouble with many women is that the guilt is hopelessly muddled with responsibility. Making sure your family is well fed is one thing, blaming yourself if they don't eat is another.

It's amazing what getting guilt out of the way can free you for. My friend Pat, a writer whose brood of children includes two teenage sons, announced she would be doing no more ironing. Finito. 'Once I was released from the tyranny of the ironing board I gained at least three hours a week. Mind you, it was hard at first to see the boys go out the door in crumpled shirts and not feel it reflected badly on me. They took a year to pick up the iron themselves, but when their holiday jobs demanded pressed white shirts they soon learnt.'

Even her husband irons his own shirts. 'He used to be so grumpy if they weren't pressed, and now he's desperately grateful if I occasionally iron a shirt for him.' Her daughters' school shirts? 'They wear them under gym slips and jumpers so why bother? I might run the iron over the collars though, and I do press their party frocks.'

Abandoning the ironing, she says, was 'extraordinarily liberating. The very thought of that basket with the clothes in it made me feel instantly tired; those hours and hours trapped at the ironing board. Now I'm free to do things I really want to do.'

If you can't face doing away with the ironing board altogether, consider handing those baskets over to an ironing service. Check your local newspaper or Yellow Pages.

But the ironing is only a fraction of it. Without thinking what is happening, working women get into the habit of taking on too much. On top of their job, they take *all* the responsibility for running the home and family. 'But my partner does the shopping,' you protest. Who makes the shopping list though? Who arranges the childminder? Who leaves instructions for the cleaning woman? Who decides what's for supper? Who puts the washing in the machine?

'Well, I prefer to do the washing. My husband and the kids are hopeless; they'll put coloureds in a hot wash so everything runs.' Or: 'I like supermarket shopping. That way I can plan our meals and make sure we don't run out of anything. I often make little impulse buys too.' Is it any wonder women are renowned in business for being appalling delegators? Are they so terrified of losing control over whatever area of authority they possess? Do they take a perverse pride in proving themselves capable? ('No one else does it better.') Or do they allow these tasks to devolve on them without question or argument, because it doesn't occur to them to do otherwise? Whichever way, too many women find themselves stretched to the limit and constantly exhausted.

At work, too, they can find it difficult to define the limits of their job, so that they shoulder bits and pieces of other people's tasks without really thinking it through. 'It's easier to do it myself.'

Sophie is a pharmacist with a national chain of chemists. She is married to Peter and they have two children. Peter runs his own business and Sophie is very conscious of the pressures and worries this means for him. The children are at secondary school so they have exams and social lives to accommodate. Sophie's elderly mother lives a few miles away and as she can't drive, Sophie pops over to keep her house clean and shops for her each week as well as herself. Her boss has just asked her to do an extra shift on Saturday mornings and she doesn't like to say no. Truth to tell, she actually feels a bit flattered. If asked why her children can't help their grandmother or do their own washing, Sophie looks astonished and concerned. This is *her* responsibility. They wouldn't do it right, and it would all have to be done again anyway.

Every now and then it all seems too much and Sophie lies down and has a little weep. Her neck aches and she has frequent headaches, because her back and shoulder muscles are so tense and hunched. She can't remember when she last read a book for pleasure. She tries to keep up by reading pharmaceutical journals in bed, but falls asleep by the second paragraph.

If Sophie is not going to land up with a stress-related illness worse than a neckache, she needs to learn some basic self-management skills: confidence building, assertiveness, and time management.

HAVE CONFIDENCE

When you lack self-confidence, pushing yourself to do anything is tiring. When you're tired, your self-confidence slips. Another self-defeating cycle – and one that happens to the most upfront and dynamic people.

Conservative MP Emma Nicholson says that when she is tired and dispirited her confidence wanes. 'Women have a greater predisposition to self-consciousness and that drains and distorts our energies. I have to stay calm inside and tell myself to get on with it.' She deflects her self-consciousness by taking her mind off herself, concentrating on others and encouraging their self-esteem.

Yet confidence is often a sham. There are huge numbers of people walking about, appearing to be in control and looking as if they can move mountains, who underneath are towers of jelly. It's a trick that men seem to pick up in the cradle from doting mothers, and women – because they were brought up to be affectionate and nurturing rather than aggressive and competitive – find harder to learn.

Inner confidence, a deep-down faith in your own worth that can send you into the world girded like Joan of Arc, is more rare. If you are not blessed with it early in life, it may require years of self-awareness and practice and sometimes therapy to acquire.

Meanwhile, behavioural psychology can help: *act* as if you are confident. That is how people will then respond to you, listening to what you have to say, assuming you know what you are talking about, and the behaviour will be reinforced. It may be tiring at first (though not as fatiguing as the impotence of not achieving what you want or deserve) but

159

one day you'll fall into it so easily you'll know it has become second nature.

'Remember that confidence starts with C-O-N,' says Liz Willis, whose training programme 'Springboard' has been followed by thousands of British women. Begin with your appearance. Much as we might gnash our teeth at the thought, first impressions *are* important. Research by American psychologist Albert Mehrabian revealed that our appearance accounts for 55 per cent of what people think about us; our voice for 35 per cent, and what we actually *say* for a mere 7 per cent. No wonder politicians spend so much time with imagemakers.

Those in the image business recommend that you identify the styles and colours that suit your personality best. Colour consultants will run you up a chart – for a fee. More challenging is deciding which style represents the True You. Much is instinctive. It cost me £85 to discover – or confirm – what I already knew in my heart: that casual but classic clothes, loose-cut, long-jacketed, are more flattering on me than frilly full skirts. Stick to what you are comfortable in, and if you're ambitious, dress for the job you want, not the one you have. Remember that if you feel good in what you're wearing, you'll look good. Your appearance will be one less thing to worry about.

Our voice is another giveaway. Nervous, gabbling, squeaky voices make mice of the most immaculately dressed men and women. Pitch your voice low and breathe from the abdomen, not high in the chest.

Tricks are all very well, but, says voice and communication expert Philippa Davies, 'however well you project your voice, or communicate succinctly, nothing will happen if inside your head you're still telling yourself "I'm weak, I'm a pushover." '

Identify those situations in which you feel most confident, and those where you feel least, and analyse why. Inner voices from our past – our mother, father, a teacher – can leave terrible scars: 'You're fat, you're stupid, you're ugly . . . You shouldn't do this; you ought to do that . . .' It's hard to ignore them, but putting names and faces to them can take away some of their power.

I know it sounds silly and toe-curlingly artificial, but telling yourself you're wonderful – what psychologists call positive affirmations – actually works. Remember the list of your assets you stuck up beside your mirror in the last chapter? Consciously remind yourself of it every day.

Occupational psychologist Ros Heaton suggests a 28-day morning and evening routine to consider: 'Five things I've achieved today; five things I'm good at; five things good about me; five things I like about my appearance; and five people who feel warmly about me.'

Confidence boosters

1. Maintain eye contact. Look at people long enough to acknowledge them and then away again.
2. Watch your body language. Confident people take up space. They don't twitch or fiddle, hunch their shoulders or cross arms and legs defensively.
3. Avoid a 'frozen' face. Tense then relax your face muscles to warm it up.
4. Take time to pause and breathe evenly.
5. If you hear your voice rising, pull it down at the end of the sentence.
6. Be prepared. Know your facts before going into a meeting, make notes for a speech.
7. Choose clothes that fit and are appropriate, so that you can forget about them.
8. Remind yourself that people have better things to do than analyse your shortcomings.
9. If you're a woman, wear lipstick.
10. Imagine yourself being successful.
11. Learn to say 'so what?' Will any of this matter in ten years' time?
12. Get a friend to give you honest feedback on your progress.

BE ASSERTIVE

Are you one of those people who sulk because your family isn't psychic and doesn't *know* that you've had a miserable day, you're premenstrual, and you want them to tidy up their mess, wash up the supper plates and tell you you're lovely? Or do you take out your frustration by flinging things around and shouting at them instead?

Or does Edna from the Parents' Association telephone to ask if you will run the tombola stall at the school fete, and you hear yourself saying yes, even though you've just taken on an extra project at work?

Women (in general and not exclusively – men aren't exempt either) can be absolutely pathetic about spelling out what they want, and play some pretty childish games as a result. Desperate to be liked by everybody, and terrified of causing a row, they let themselves fall into the fatigue trap because they can't – or won't – ask for help, and they take on too much because they can't – or won't – say no.

Anne Dickson, whose book *A Woman In Your Own Right – Assertiveness and You* is still the classic textbook on the subject, says there are three essential skills to be learnt.

1. Decide what it is you want or feel, and say so – specifically and directly.
2. Stick to your statement, repeating it, if necessary, over and over again.
3. Deflect any responses that might undermine your position.

For example, you've come home exhausted from a beastly day at the office and the kids have left dirty plates in the sink and a constellation of coffee mugs in the sitting room, where your partner is ensconced with his feet up, reading the newspaper and ignoring the mess.

The Assertive You says 'I'm tired and I'd like you all to help me get supper ready. I'd like you (the children) to wash up your plates and mugs and I'd like you (your partner) to lay the table.'

They may be so astonished at this clear request that they comply – or they may ignore you or argue. No problem. Calmly, you repeat your statement. Someone will try to deflect you, perhaps. 'I've been in a frightful meeting all afternoon,' says your husband. 'We've got homework,' say the children. Does this bother you? No. 'I'm sorry about your meeting,' you say, 'and there's plenty of time for homework. I'd like you to wash up and lay the table.' Refrain from getting vicious, as in 'If you want any bloody supper, you'd better do what I ask.' They are not stupid; they will eventually get the message. And you haven't lost your temper and frazzled yourself even more.

Practice will make perfect.

Saying 'No'

If you say 'no' to a request you are not necessarily being: selfish, callous, mean, small-minded, churlish, rude, aggressive, hurtful. Remember this.

When someone asks you to do something, suggests Anne Dickson, *notice your immediate reaction*. The first thought in your mind may be 'yes', in which case accept. If it's 'no', then refuse – and stick to your refusal, no matter what blandishments or coercion are offered. If you can't decipher a message from your inner self, then *ask for more information*.

You can stall and say you need to think about it. Or, if it's Edna about the tombola, ask 'what would I have to do?' Find out exactly what is involved so that you can make up your mind.

If you are going to say no, then don't mess about overelaborating your excuses. An explanation is fine, so long as you genuinely want to give a reason for your refusal, and aren't worrying that you'll be thought selfish, callous and all the rest of it, or feeling guilty about letting someone down.

Practise saying 'No.' Just like that. 'No.' 'When you say "no",' says Anne Dickson, 'you are refusing the request, not rejecting the person.'

Other tips

★ Give the other person an opportunity to express their feelings, so that they don't feel completely rejected by your refusal.

★ On the other hand, don't hang around making stilted conversation simply because you feel embarrassed and want to appear friendly – the refusee probably wants to move on and ask somebody else.

★ Offer a compromise if it's appropriate.

★ If you feel awkward, don't be afraid to admit it: 'I find this difficult' allows both of you a chance to express your feelings.

So, Edna, I'm going to say no to organising the tombola. I have a very full workload at the moment and I couldn't put the necessary time into it. However, I would be happy to help out on the day of the fete.

There.

MAKING TIME

Time management means getting some control over the haphazard hours of the day; the minutes that run away; the seconds that slide off heaven knows where. Men often seem enviably better at organising their time than women, but their lives are also usually less fractured by fiddly activities and responsibilities. Rightly or wrongly, they don't sit in conferences wondering if they'll have a chance to slip out and re-organise the school run.

In theory, if you could control your time, you'd be in control of your life. You wouldn't be taking work home because you were interrupted a zillion times during the day. You could schedule workout sessions twice a week and not waste lunch hours shopping for food. You'd arrive on cue for meetings and you'd allow enough time to get from A to B. ('Harry is always late,' says his wife, 'because when he says he'll be there at three, what he really means is that he's leaving at three. He forgets about the ten minutes travelling.') You'd have time to go to the cinema and get eight hours' sleep. You'd have time to make love and not always be complaining you're too tired.

So what do you do? Being assertive and saying no are part of it. Deciding what is important to you is another.

An American psychologist studied top performing people in all walks of life and discovered they shared certain characteristics. They weren't, as you might expect, workaholics who were driven by a fear of failure and at the mercy of fatigue. They were motivated – energised – by goals they had set themselves.

They didn't skimp holidays because they couldn't 'afford' the time for them, but used them for rest and creative thinking.

They delegated like mad, assigning any tasks that could be done by other people, and avoiding those seductive but time-consuming projects that lead nowhere. And they didn't try to be perfect.

Endless books are written on time management, because people who need to control their time prefer to think about it rather than actually do it. There's even an element of resistance: I haven't *time* to stop and organise myself. In fact, the rules are really very basic.

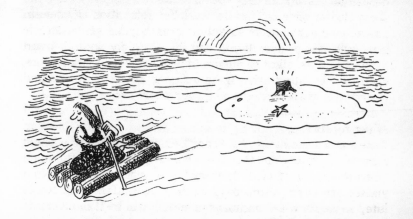

1. Set aside a period of planning for the week ahead, checking that appointments don't clash and allocating time for particular tasks.

2. Ask yourself do I need to do this job myself, or can I pass it on to someone else?

3. Each day allow at least ten minutes' planning time.

4. Make a daily To Do list. Everyone has their own idiosyncratic way of doing this: A lists and B lists; work lists and personal lists; absolutely urgent, do at once, and do one day when there's nothing else lists. However you structure it, mark those items which must be done today and which can wait, and tick off each item as it's completed. This is very cheering and nothing is more satisfying than a row of ticks by lunch time.

5. Allow only a certain time for routine chores. I could file papers and cuttings until the cows come home, but it wouldn't help me meet deadlines. More effective would be half an hour's 'housekeeping' every day.

6. Make yourself unavailable if you have something that must be finished without interruptions. Shut the door, put your telephone answering machine on. If you are interrupted, tell the caller you will ring back in half an hour, three hours, or whatever, when you will have time to talk (and make sure that you do).

7. Slot in several hours a week for relaxation. Remember that your time is as valuable as anyone else's, and by nurturing yourself you will have the energy to nurture others. It might sound daft, but if you would like to spend two or three evenings reading a novel or listening to music then set it down on your weekly schedule.

Sharing time

There is no correlation between the number of years a couple has been together and the amount of time they spend talking to each other – in fact, it is probably a declining ratio. When people are busy, wrapped up in their own affairs, the person they share their bed and mortgage with can be taken as much for granted. Alison described her husband Jim as becoming as familiar as the wallpaper. 'We communicated in a language of marital grunts. Would he be in for supper? Uhh-hhhh. Had he seen the television programme? Nnng-nnnn.'

The children, your colleagues, your friends, your aged parents, even the dog, can have first claim on your attention, and the result is that time spent on nurturing and growing your relationship is lost. You forget to talk. Worse, you can forget *how* to talk to each other.

'We crawl into bed, too exhausted for anything as strenuous as sex,' says one woman. 'If we do make love, then it's over in seconds – a "quickie". Often all I want is a cuddle, but if I make an affectionate approach, my husband takes it as a green light for sex. So we end up hardly touching each other.'

The irony (and the tragedy) is that, if only she could have shared her feelings with her partner, a cuddle, a loving empathetic hug, would have done so much to revive her tired spirit. Instead she expends energy lying rigid in bed, for fear that she might inadvertently arouse him.

Good communication is so often the key to any relationship problem. By and large, we are not blessed with clairvoyance, and if you express your fatigue and frustration by sulking, shouting, nagging or picking arguments over other minor issues, then it's very difficult to stop and think, 'Ah yes, poor Fred, he's blaming me for supper not being ready because he's shortstaffed, his secretary's sick and he has to make somebody redundant tomorrow.'

If you would appreciate more help in the house – or more tolerance and understanding about work pressures, or support with the children – then discuss it with your partner. Curiously, vital but personally touchy subjects such as sex or household responsibilities, ones loaded with critical implications for both of you, can be exactly those that are most difficult to broach.

But what's the point playing the martyr if nobody knows you're suffering? A husband may not rush to volunteer with the washing up, but equally he may not realise what a load his wife is carrying. He certainly won't unless she tells him, and asks for help.

Studies around the world show that working women spend more time in housework and less on leisure than men. But where's the New Man? you ask. The partner who shares all, the dirty nappies, cleaning the loo, getting up to crying kids at night. As far as most people are concerned, he's a myth, a mirage.

To be scrupulously fair, men under 40 are certainly readier to lend a hand than those a generation older, who grew up in the bad old days when chaps were chaps and wouldn't be seen dead wheeling a pram to the supermarket. But social revolutions are numbingly slow. I suspect it will be several decades yet before the majority of husbands and partners really share roles, taking it in turns to cook dinner and stay home from work to mind sick children. And it won't happen unless women insist on their co-operation.

Part of the secret lies in getting in first, when you first set up home together before the children arrive, and hammering out who will do what. But the other, most important part is keeping the channels of communication open, continuing to talk about those things that are profoundly important to you – your dreams, ambitions, fears – and not just the practical will-you-be-home-for-dinner-have-you-fixed-the-sink matters.

How can you do this when you're both rushing around in separate worlds? Build time into the week when you put other distractions aside and sit down and talk. Invest in a babysitter and go out for dinner, perhaps. Take a long walk. Put the children to bed and turn off the television.

And then what do you say? According to Relate, the national marriage guidance council, the essence of good communication can be summed up in three points.

1. Say exactly how you feel.
2. Listen to what the other says.
3. Accept your partner's opinions and feelings even when they're different from your own.

We all fall into bad habits and manipulative tricks when dealing with other people. Now's the time to remember your assertiveness guidelines.

Say what you really mean.
If your partner always accepts an invitation to Sunday lunch with his parents, and you're fed up with never being consulted and anyway, you want to do something else at the weekend, then explain – calmly, reasonably – how you feel. You could say 'I know you like to see your parents, but sometimes I feel very tired and I'd like to spend the day at home reading the papers. Why don't you lunch with them by yourself this week – I'm sure they'd like to see you on your own.' *Don't* say (even if it's what you feel) 'I'm sick to death of your bloody mother and father every weekend, you can tell them to stuff it, I'm spending the day in bed.'

Don't fudge.
People complain about trivial issues to avoid talking about the big problem. It's not the fact that he drops his clothes on the floor; it's that he never *ever* picks anything up and expects you to keep the house tidy even though you both go out to work.

Don't nag.
Telling someone what you think should be done – or not done – over and over again isn't helpful communication. Anyway, they switch off, and all the energy you've put into nagging them is wasted.

Listen.
This is one of the hardest things to do. It means giving someone all your attention, so that they feel what they're saying is important and worthwhile. It means not interrupting (men are dreadful about this). It means not jumping in with your own point of view as soon as someone finishes talking. It means not changing the subject. It means putting your own thoughts aside and really trying to understand the other person. All this

can be quite tiring, but it will be an effort worth making because the rewards will be great.

References

Personal Power by Philippa Davies (Piatkus)
The Relate Guide to Better Relationships by Sarah Litvinoff (Ebury Press)
The Superwoman Syndrome by Marjorie Shaevitz (Fontana)
Your Total Image by Philippa Davies (Piatkus)
A Woman In Your Own Right – Assertiveness And You by Anne Dickson (Quartet Books)

Relate,
 Herbert Gray College,
 Little Church Street,
 Rugby CV21 3AP
 (tel. 0788 573241)

CHAPTER 12

Release your healing resources

JUST DO IT!

Have you ever been in the middle of a crowd of people? It's difficult – and even frightening – when you're being jostled on all sides, to see where you're going or how many people there actually are. But if you climbed a tree or a ladder, the perspective would be quite different. You could still physically identify with the crowd, but your view of what was happening would be detached and more informed.

In the same way it can be dreadfully hard to make sense of your life when you're down there in the melee (figuratively speaking), being shoved back and forth by conflicting pressures and growing tired and dispirited and panicky. What you want is a tree (aha!) to take you above it all and give you an overall impression of the situation; a feeling of control that keeps you one step ahead of fatigue.

Going away on holidays and long weekends and retreats are valuable, but you can't disappear like that every day. A 'tree' could be a means of taking you out of your everyday self, that would allow your mind and body to integrate so the healing resources of one can influence the other.

Here is the happy news: there are techniques and therapies available that can act as 'trees'. Some work on the body, unknotting tense muscles and releasing a cascade of endorphins and other hormones that can relax and soothe you. Others tap the power of the mind to slow the heartbeat and respiration and induce the slow smooth brainwaves of tranquillity and well-being.

The easiest – in the sense that you don't have to do anything except lie there and be done to – are the body therapies: massage and healing. There's no escaping the fact that they will cost you money – the average hourly fee for an aromatherapist, for example, is £20–£30 – but it can be a very worthwhile investment.

Maybe it's because of growing up with the National Health Service, which is wonderful when you're really ill, but the British can be notoriously mean about shelling out money on their health – especially when they aren't even *sick*. Yet, as June, a massage therapist, comments to clients wriggling at her fees, 'How much do you spend on maintaining your car in a year?'

If people would only maintain themselves better, she insists, following de-stressing therapies while in good health, they would handle pressures better when they happen and feel less tired and depressed. 'We have people who know they have crazy schedules and come in regularly to keep themselves finely tuned. That way there's less stress on their system and they can not only cope with their work, but enjoy it too.'

MASSAGE

Another thing the British have always been a bit funny about is touching each other – i.e., they don't – so the idea of somebody running their hands over you while you lie there and enjoy it strikes a lot of people as somehow self-indulgent and decadent. Unfortunately there are also unhelpful connotations with massage parlours and the last place to look for a masseuse is usually the Yellow Pages.

Massage is one of the oldest healing tools. Hippocrates, the Father of Medicine (he whose oath doctors take) wrote in the 5th century BC: 'The way to health is to have a scented bath and an oiled massage each day.'

In the hands of a qualified therapist, it's an excellent way of relaxing both mind and body. Blood flows more freely, waste products are swept away from muscle cells, aches and pains are eased, and depression lifts. After a good massage, people fraught with anxiety find they can handle worries more constructively and self-confidently.

As one fortunate enough to have received a massage from Clare Maxwell-Hudson, the doyenne of Britain's massage therapists, I'll vouch for all that. You step off the couch feeling inexpressibly calm and somehow revitalised at the same time. Old Hippocrates knew what he was on about.

Massage therapy is now taught to third-year students at the Royal College of Nursing, and in hospitals like Charing Cross, London, nurses have used it to bring down patients' blood pressure before and after operations. Touch, and the empathy and compassion that accompany it, are taken very seriously as healing aids in many sections of the medical profession.

Massage has the bonus of making the therapist feel better too: using touch to help someone else evokes a very personal sense of mutual trust. You don't have to be qualified to discover this – Clare Maxwell-Hudson's *The Complete Book of Massage* will give you enough hints to practise soothing strokes on a friend or partner.

References

The Clare Maxwell-Hudson School of Massage,
  PO Box 457,
  London NW2 4BR
  (tel. 081-450 6494)

The London College of Massage,
  5-6 Newman Passage,
  London W1P 3PF
  (tel. 071-323 3574)

The Complete Book of Massage by Clare Maxwell-Hudson
  (Dorling Kindersley)

Aromatherapy massage
It's tempting to describe this as massage with smells. However, the smells are the important bit, and the massage is a nice way of getting them on and into the body. The smells, in fact, are those of plant extracts – called essences or essential oils – which are believed to have healing properties when absorbed into the system through the skin. (See Chapter 3)

Particular smells have been shown to have an immediate effect on the brain, and an aromatherapy massage is a pretty heady experience. The effects can be either deeply soothing or stimulating, depending on the oil used, so make sure you tell the therapist how you want to feel.

Aromatherapy has a delicious element of the exotic about it. The ancient Egyptians practised it – scent pots were found in Tutankhamun's tomb – and the oils themselves were wonderfully romantic: it takes 2,000 pounds or rose petals to produce one ounce of rose oil.

In massage, the essences are diluted in a 'carrier' of vegetable oil or alcohol. Concentrated essential oils are too strong to put directly on the skin or to swallow, unless advised by a trained aromatherapist, but you can absorb them safely by adding a few drops to the bath or inhaling them from a tissue.

If you're tempted to use aromatherapy at home, there are short courses and workshops which teach the basics, although a professional aromatherapist studies up to 12 months for a diploma.

References

International Federation of Aromatherapists,
  Department of Continuing Education,
  Royal Masonic Hospital,
  Ravenscourt Park,
  London W6 0TN
  (tel. 081-846 8066)

Aromatherapy Organisations Council,
  3 Latymer Close,
  Braybrooke,
  Market Harborough,
  Leics. LE16 8LN

Shiatsu

Rather more bracing than body massage (you are less likely to nod off) shiatsu is an ancient Japanese massage that uses pressure on the body's acupuncture points to stimulate the flow of *Qi* or life force through the meridians (energy paths). Shiatsu means 'finger massage', but the therapist's palm and heel of the hand, elbow, forearm, knee, foot, and especially the thumbs come into it too.

If you can't swallow *Qi*, one theory has it that shiatsu rebalances subtle electromagnetic forces in the body. Whatever the explanation, shiatsu practitioners seem able to make you feel either elated or sedated, depending on which meridians they work with, and they'll usually spend some time asking you about your general health before embarking on the massage.

A businessman who travels to the Far East several times a year always treats himself to a massage at the shiatsu headquarters in Tokyo. 'It's a real shot in the arm. I go in tired and tense and jetlagged and come away invigorated,' he says.

Fortunately there are plenty of shiatsu practitioners in Britain, who have great success in treating general fatigue, stress, tension, depression, insomnia, headaches and backpain. As preventive medicine, shiatsu is an excellent tonic for the whole body, mind and spirit that can boost the immune system. And unlike body massage, you keep your clothes on – wear something loose-fitting and comfortable.

Fiona was dragging herself into work, frayed with stress and anxiety, when she started a course of shiatsu, a fortnightly massage for six months. 'I had huge knots of tension in my shoulders and I could feel them going with each massage. I feel so much better. I'm now convinced that it's vital to recognise when you're using up your energy reserves and do something before you get really sick.'

Do-in is a form of do-it-yourself shiatsu, useful first thing in the morning to make you more energetic, and at any time of the day to relieve stress and improve concentration. It's best learned from a shiatsu practitioner, to make sure you're on the right road.

Reference

The Shiatsu Society,
   5 Foxcote,
   Wokingham,
   Berkshire RG1 3PG
   (tel. 0734 730836).

REFLEXOLOGY

Explaining how and why massaging your big toe can relieve tension strains a brain raised on Western science, but any number of people swear by reflexology. According to the theory, the organs and systems of the body are 'reflected' in different areas of your foot. The heart, for example, is somewhere near the ball of the foot; the small intestine nearer the heel. Like acupuncture and shiatsu, it's based on the ancient Chinese concept of energy pathways connecting every part of the body and terminating in the feet, hands and head.

A couple of years ago a group of NHS nurses in Manchester experimented with reflexology to relieve anxiety amongst elderly people. Those receiving reflexology reported greater drops in anxiety than a control group receiving counselling, and those receiving ordinary nursing were, if anything, even more anxious.

If nothing else, it's very soothing and leaves you with an exquisite sense of well-being.

References

British Reflexology Association,
  Monks Orchard,
  Whitbourne,
  Worcester WR6 5RB
  (Send £1.50 for a list of qualified private practitioners.)

The British School of Reflexology,
  92 Sheering Road,
  Old Harlow,
  Essex CM17 0JW
  (tel. 0279 429060)

FLOTATION

You float gently in about a foot of water in total or semi-darkness and silence. The water is skin temperature (about 34.2°C) and filled with Epsom salts and other minerals to keep you buoyant. And there you are, for anything from one to two and a half hours, with nothing between you and your thoughts. The idea is that without sensory distractions you can concentrate on the inner self, roam through your imagination and listen to the mental and biological voices of the body. In such a womb-like state, some experts believe, you learn to control physiological systems such as blood pressure and even enhance the immune system. Maybe.

Those who have tried it, however, report a calming experience. 'I thought I'd be claustrophobic and bored,' said Felicity, 'but I came out feeling as you do when you first wake up in the morning, before you start worrying about what to wear or whether you'll catch the bus.'

Practitioners recommend it for anyone suffering from fatigue, stress and anxiety – though not deep depression. You can escape if you can't stand it any longer; the door to the tank is always unlocked.

Reference

Flotation Tank Association,
  29 Sunbury Lane,
  London SW11 3NP

Body therapies, such as those above, are very restful, in that you lie there and let the practitioner do all the work. Others, however, engage the mind and require learning. There is an initial outlay for classes, but after that you are on your own, and theoretically able to practise on yourself.

ALEXANDER TECHNIQUE

Standing and sitting badly is a bigger cause of fatigue than we realise. Hunch your shoulders, slump in a chair, twist your spine, and you're pulling muscles and nerves out of alignment, squeezing your internal organs, and breathing badly. The Alexander Technique teaches you to be aware of your posture, and to move in a co-ordinated way so that your body can relax and work more naturally and efficiently.

A course can be anything from 12 to 30 lessons, depending on how well you relearn to hold yourself. The teacher begins by watching how you use your body – walking, sitting, standing – and then stretches you out on a couch and tweaks at your arms and legs, adjusts your head and spine and stands you up and says 'Look at the difference.' This is usually so astonishing – I felt at least two inches taller and I rediscovered my neck and chin – that you are motivated to reproduce the same effect yourself.

The key is a series of instructions or 'orders' which you practise until they are second nature: free the neck, head forward and up, back long and wide. Ultimately, however, the effectiveness of the Technique is up to you and how much you follow it in your everyday life.

There's no doubt that balancing the body has a knock-on

effect on the mind. I felt calmer and more in control, but it also started me thinking and feeling in new ways, about how my life could be less tiring and better ordered.

Reference

The Society of Teachers of the Alexander Technique,
   20 London House,
   266 Fulham Road,
   London SW10 9EL
   (tel. 071-351 0828)

AUTOGENIC TRAINING

Sceptical business executives are usually comfortable with this therapy. There's no funny philosophy behind it, you don't have to get undressed, and it's all perfectly sensible and scientific. In fact, it's usually taught by doctors, nurses, psychologists and other health workers, and absolutely normal people like airline pilots learn it to overcome jet lag.

Autogenic training is a method of achieving deep relaxation, in which the body is able to free its own healing processes and maintain well-being. Under guidance, you learn a series of simple mental exercises, repeating to yourself such phrases as 'my right arm is heavy', 'my left leg is warm', that will induce this relaxed state.

A course usually consists of about eight or ten ninety-minute sessions in a small group. Once mastered, you can practise the technique at will, whenever and wherever you wish. People who use it say they have better concentration, more energy and are less affected by stress.

Reference

Centre for Autogenic Training,
   Positive Health Centre,

101 Harley Street,
London W1N 1DF
(tel. 071-935 1811)

COLOUR THERAPY

American psychologists were riveted to discover that prisoners became calmer and more amenable when their cell walls were painted a particular shade of pink that exactly matched the lining of the womb. Nobody's advocating a mass regression for the rest of us, but we're probably well aware that certain colours affect our mood and concentration and even reflect our personality. We feel 'blue', go 'white' with fright, and 'green' with jealousy.

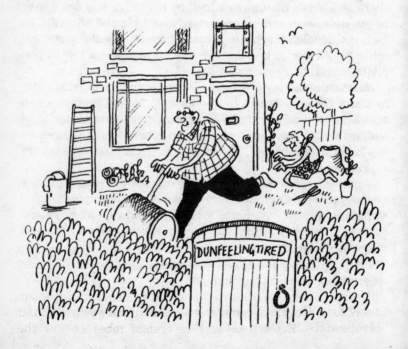

Colour therapists believe that the body absorbs the various electromagnetic wavelengths of light and emits an aura of its own, the colours of which will reflect your current emotional, spiritual and physical health. Treatment involves being bathed in different coloured lights – lack of energy, depression and stress are said to be alleviated by this.

More practically, using particular colours in your clothes and your environment can enhance a certain state of mind. Red, orange and yellow are all colours of vitality and energy – but painting a room red could be rather overwhelming. Use them with discretion. Turquoise, which inspires feelings of freshness and aliveness, is said to work well in studies and office areas.

References

The International Association for Colour Therapy,
  73 Elm Bank Gardens,
  Barnes,
  London SW13 0NX

The Hygeia College of Colour Therapy,
  Theo Gimbel,
  Brook House,
  Avening,
  Tetbury,
  Gloucs. GL8 8NS
  (tel. 045 383 2150)

MEDITATION

Once learned and practised, meditation is the supreme self-help remedy, inducing at once an inner calm and a brimming focus of energy that overcomes fatigue.

Unfortunately, the practice has had a rather cranky press in the West. A lot of people see it as a peculiar and awkward habit advocated by Eastern mystics in orange robes and by the followers of the Maharishi Mahesh Yogi, who teach Transcendental Meditation and occasionally appear in levitational attitudes in the tabloids.

What is often forgotten is that meditation has been practised by Christian orders for centuries – the spiritual exercises of St Ignatius Loyola, founder of the Jesuits, include many meditational techniques. Mantras – words or formulas repeated to clear the mind – have been used by Christians ('Kyrie eleison' – 'Lord have mercy' is an old favourite) as well as Buddhists ('Om'), Sufis, Yogis, and Hasidic Jews.

You don't have to be religious to meditate, nor will you become woolly and otherworldly. Rather the opposite. People who meditate regularly not only seem to have a zest and gusto for life, but are extraordinarily efficient at what they do for a living. Those who have followed it for many years report moments of profound bliss and fulfilment.

Physiologically the benefits are remarkable. The heartbeat slows, blood pressure and respiration rates decrease and the metabolic rate is lowered. The brain wave pattern changes to long alpha waves that are a sign of deep relaxation coupled with a state of mental alertness.

Sitting about cross-legged with your eyes shut looks easy but the discipline requires rigorous mental effort and application and it is important to find the method that suits you best. Some schools of meditation can be dogmatic about insisting that their way is the only one to follow.

The aim is to concentrate your mind on one object, and one object only, to the exclusion of everything else. Repeating mantras is only one way to achieve this. You could equally contemplate a picture, observe your thought, follow your breathing, practise T'ai Chi (see Chapter 9) – an active form of meditation – or even arrange flowers. Don't confuse it with pleasant but flabby daydreaming – your will must be actively engaged in keeping your focus on the meditation.

People do manage successfully, but it can be quite hard to start meditating on your own. Find a group if possible. The local library might be able to help.

How to meditate

1. Find a place where you won't be disturbed for at least twenty minutes. You might want to set an alarm clock or timer so you are not distracted by thoughts of 'how much longer?' Turn off the radio, take the telephone off the hook.
2. Make sure the room is warm and your clothes comfortable.
3. Don't meditate within two hours after a meal. You will derive most benefit if you practise for fifteen or twenty minutes twice a day, before breakfast and before supper.
4. A cross-legged lotus pose isn't necessary. Sit on an upright chair, your back comfortably straight, feet firmly on the ground, and your hands in your lap or on your knees, palms either up or down. Align the tip of your nose with your navel. Close your eyes and relax. Let yourself *be*.
5. Breathe rhythmically and slowly through your nose and down into your abdomen.
6. Concentrate absolutely single-mindedly on the object of your meditation. It could be your breath, watching it go out, go in, as you count to four. It might be a flower, an image, or a word or phrase. Even a nonsense word will do, although some people use 'Peace' or 'Love one another'.
7. Don't panic if your mind wanders, or all kinds of distracting thoughts buzz into your head. You can find yourself planning the report you have to write, wondering about supper, or even thinking 'am I doing this okay?' Just gently but firmly bring your concentration back, again and again, to the object of meditation.
8. That's all, really. On the first occasion you will feel self-conscious and it may not seem very successful. Keep practising and you will begin to understand why some people think of meditation as dipping into a deep and refreshing well.

References

How To Meditate by Lawrence LeShan (Thorsons)
Introducing Meditation by Dr Sarah Eagger (tape and booklet)
  from the
British Holistic Medical Association,
  179 Gloucester Place,
  London NW1 6DX
  (tel. 071-262 5299)

BIOFEEDBACK

What next? A mind-controlled computer programme, Relax-
Plus, is now available that teaches you to relax at home. First
developed at St Bartholomew's Hospital, London, there are two
sensor pads for your fingers that measure tiny fluctuations in
blood flow and sweat and are linked to the images on the
screen. Most fun is a game, Evolve, in which – if you relax
enough – a fish turns into a mermaid who swims to an island
and becomes an angel flying into the sky and eventually a star.
One twitch, however, and you'll find yourself back in the briny.

The package also includes scientifically devised self-
monitoring programmes that can train you so efficiently that
you consciously induce relaxation in seconds.

RelaxPlus can be used with any IBM compatible computer
with a colour screen and a mouse. Price £189 from Ultramind.

Reference

Ultramind,
  5 Ravenscroft Avenue,
  London NW11 0SA
  (tel. 071-982 6092)

CHAPTER 13

All in the mind

FEELING BLUE

There are misery-making, brain-churning, exhausting states of mind that drain your physical and mental energy as efficiently as if you'd left a tap running. Stress may trigger them, or exacerbate them, but once you are in their grip, spiralling down in depression, or tortured by anxiety, your vigour, your creativity and your zest for life will be wrung out of you.

The most pervasive, the most serious, is depression. In one degree or another, it can accompany other conditions – loneliness, bereavement, anxiety – as naturally as butter goes on bread, and yet its presence is so insidious that you may not recognise it as the cause of your fatigue and hopelessness.

But beware jumping to conclusions: tiredness *in itself* doesn't mean you are on the verge of a breakdown. Lack of sleep and pressure from work and family makes us all fed up and 'down' at times. 'Life doesn't seem worth living,' complained Hilary, a young working mother. 'I'm up to the baby twice a night, and we can't get Zoë, the toddler, to go to sleep until all hours. Then I have to be out of bed at six thirty. I drag myself into the office and I push myself through the day. I can't concentrate; I can't work up any enthusiasm for anything. I feel so depressed.'

A week later, when the baby finishes teething, and she and her husband have left the children with their grandmother and spent a weekend with friends in the country, Hilary is a sparkling new woman. Her depression has evaporated like a cloud in the sun.

It wouldn't be the first time tiredness has been mistaken for depression. A man complained that he was depressed to psychologists Susan Tanner and Jillian Ball. He woke with a dull headache, he claimed, and lacked motivation for anything. 'When we questioned him more closely, we discovered that he had worked overtime several nights during the week and had been out socialising until early that morning, so he had good reason to be tired.' They pointed out that his symptoms were due to exhaustion rather than depression, and his spirits immediately lifted. Thank you, he said, he felt much better.

The moral of this? Don't talk yourself into a gloom unnecessarily without looking for a simpler explanation. Having said that, however, many people *are* genuinely depressed, but are unaware of it, or prefer to think they are suffering from something else. Dr Susan Abbey, one of the world's leading experts in Chronic Fatigue Syndrome (known in Britain as ME), is blunt. 'Among women in the age range of 20 to 50, the most likely cause of profound fatigue is depression,' she says. 'The second most likely cause is depression. And the third is depression.'

A kind of low-level depression can sap energy levels over months and years, while causing vague aches and pains. Sufferers feel 'blah' most of the time, according to psychiatrist Dr Mark Rapaport. 'They feel chronically tired. It's as if they are always looking at the world through dark glasses. Nothing ever feels terribly good. Many people with this disorder are looking for an explanation why they feel bad, and one explanation they can identify with is Chronic Fatigue Syndrome.'

There's a danger here, because their affliction is not CFS (or ME), and the sufferer struggles on in a twilight world when there are any number of effective treatments available for depression – and especially the kind of mild or moderate depression that is not instantly recognisable – if only they knew how to ask for help.

Because of an absurd and outdated stigma attached to mental illness, many men and women are still embarrassed or ashamed to confide in their GP, let alone their friends or relatives. And yet in psychiatric terms, depression is the equivalent of the common cold. Five per cent of the adult population of Britain, or two million adults, suffer from it at any one time, including comedian Spike Milligan and cartoonist Mel Calman. Nearly a third of all Britons will experience what Winston Churchill called his 'black dog' at some stage in their lifetime. Two out of three sufferers are women and only half of all victims seek professional help.

What does depression feel like? 'There is this terrible emptiness,' says Spike Milligan. 'It is like every fibre in your body is screaming for relief yet there is no relief.' Others talk of being at the bottom of a black pit or lost in a tunnel; a terrible, paralysing sense of isolation.

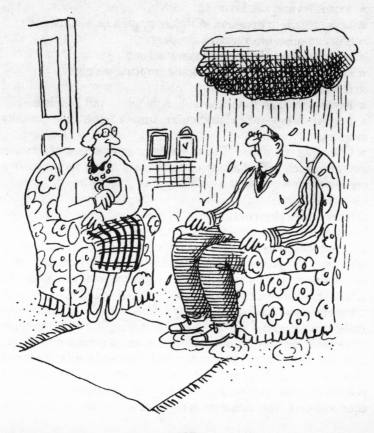

The Royal College of Psychiatrists and the Royal College of General Practitioners, who launched a five-year campaign, Defeat Depression, in 1993, list the following symptoms of major depression. If at least four apply to you, and have done for two weeks or more despite all your efforts to lift yourself out of the trough, then make an appointment to see your GP.

★ A loss of interest and enjoyment in life.
★ A lack of drive and motivation, that makes even simple tasks and decisions difficult or impossible.
★ Utter fatigue.
★ Agitation and restlessness.
★ Loss or gain in appetite, with loss or gain in weight.
★ Sleeplessness or excessive sleeping.
★ Loss of outward affection; going off sex.
★ Loss of self-confidence; avoiding meeting people.
★ Irritability.
★ Feeling useless, inadequate, bad, helpless and hopeless.
★ Feeling worse at a particular time of the day, usually mornings.
★ Thoughts of suicide. These are very common in depression and are much better admitted than covered up, as they are a certain sign that help is needed.

What causes depression?
Psychologists and psychiatrists indulge in heated arguments over whether depression is genetic and can be inherited, or whether it's psychological and due to your parents being beastly when you were a child, or whether it's social and can be blamed on life events like divorce or losing your job.

Psychologist Dr Dorothy Rowe, for example, whose books *Beyond Fear*, and *The Depression Handbook* have illuminated the lives of thousands of people, adamantly rejects any claims that depression could be genetic. But psychiatrist Dr Anthony Clare believes that the truth is probably a combination of factors – genes, personality, stress, upbringing, environment – that will vary from one person to another.

One in ten women, for instance, suffers from post-natal depression (something more persistent and crippling than the 'baby blues'). The fact that more women than men are depressed has a lot to do with the struggle to reconcile a job and a family, or being trapped at home alone with small children. But when it comes to manic depression, a condition in which moods swing from elation to suicidal despair and has clear genetic links, then there's little to choose between the sexes.

According to a new and exciting theory, depression could result when, or if, all the trigger factors come together in the brain in such a way that our biological clock is disrupted. Dr Clare describes this as 'the overriding control mechanism regulating our waking and sleeping, our activity and our relaxing, our drive and our rest,' and it could explain some symptoms of depression such as waking up at 3 a.m., losing your appetite and feeling tired and debilitated and hopeless.

It also looks as if communication between brain cells is impaired in a large number of severely depressed patients (i.e. people who can't function normally – get up and go to work or look after their children). In the usual way of things, information whizzes around the brain and to other parts of the body and back again via electrical impulses. These jump from one cell to the next with the help of chemical messengers, or neurotransmitters, such as noradrenalin and serotonin.

Antidepressants are very good at improving the function of ailing neurotransmitters, especially a new breed of drug known as selective 5-HT re-uptake inhibitors (*not* a name to remember easily). Trade names include Faverin, Seroxat, Lustral – and the popular Prozac, already seen as a kind of wonder drug that can transform a doomy pessimist into a confident optimist.

These have fewer side effects than the traditional trycyclic antidepressants – though they can still provoke nausea, drowsiness, insomnia and 'the jitters' – and are harder to overdose on, but they are more expensive. Unlike tranquillisers, which some GPs still prescribe rather futilely for depression, the new drugs are not addictive – but some psychiatrists are alarmed at the number of doctors who hand them out routinely to anybody tripping into their surgery complaining that they feel depressed, without offering counselling or psychotherapy as well.

Psychiatrists say that most patients respond to a double-pronged approach of antidepressants and psychotherapy, but that drugs may not be needed at all. For someone who is mildly to moderately depressed, due to stress or a life crisis, a little counselling – even a judicious bit of self-help – might be enough to pull them out of the Slough of Despond.

How to help yourself

★ Don't bottle things up. If something awful has happened to you – you've been made redundant, your mother has died, even a row with a colleague – tell somebody close to you about it. Relive the experience, have a good cry. Too many Britons are brought up with a stiff upper lip and a misplaced sense of dignity, but talking things through is healthy and natural, and part of the mind's way of healing itself.

★ Do something. This is particularly true for anybody crushed by fatigue or lack of concentration who feels that even crawling out of bed is too much effort. Get out of the house, go for a walk, clean out a cupboard, make a cake – anything to take your mind off the painful feelings that threaten to swamp you. You might also feel a little less helpless (and the family will enjoy the cake).

★ Eat a good balanced diet. (See Chapter 8.)

★ Resist the temptation to drown your sorrows in drink. Alcohol might give temporary relief but you'll end up feeling worse.

★ Don't get yourself worked up about not sleeping. Listen to the radio or watch television rather than lying in despair. (See Chapter 7.)

★ Remind yourself that you are suffering from depression. Many other people have been down this road, maybe even further than you, and they eventually came out into the sunshine, just as you will – however impossible that seems at the moment. This experience could even have a silver lining: you will be stronger and wiser, better able to cope than before and to take important decisions about your life. Tell yourself that you are All Right; you are a good and valuable person.

If you know someone who is depressed
Always take seriously any comments they make about not wanting to live, or wanting to hurt themselves. Insist that their doctor is told. If you have any doubts about the treatment, discuss them with the doctor, not with the sufferer.

Spend time with them, listen, encourage and reassure them.

References

Association for Post-Natal Illness,
 25 Jerdan Place,
 London SW6 1BE
 (tel. 071-386 0868)

The Defeat Depression Campaign,
 The Royal College of Psychiatrists,
 17 Belgrave Square,
 London SW1X 8PG

Depressives Anonymous,
 36 Chestnut Avenue,
 Beverley,
 Humberside HU17 9QU
 (tel. 0482 860619)

Depressives Associated,
 PO Box 1022,
 London SE1 7QB
 (tel. 081-760 0544)

MIND,
  National Association for Mental Health,
  22 Harley Street,
  London W1N 2ED
  (tel. 071-637 0741)

The Samaritans
  (see your telephone directory for your local branch)

Beating the Blues by Susan Tanner and Jillian Ball (Sheldon)
Beyond Fear by Dorothy Rowe (Fontana)
The Depression Handbook by Dorothy Rowe (Collins)
Depression and How To Survive It by Spike Milligan and
  Anthony Clare (Ebury)

GRIEF

Loss – whether it's a partner to another lover, a friend or a
parent to death, your job, your home, a limb – opens the
floodgates of emotion in a way you would not have thought
possible. All kinds of complicated and seemingly inappropriate
feelings are stirred up and spilled out – or, worse, pushed back
and fenced in.

Those who have been bereaved are alarmed to discover the
violence of their anger and guilt over the dead. 'What right did
he have to go and die and leave me like this,' railed a widow
when her husband died of cancer.

'I never had a chance to say goodbye; to tell her I really loved
her and I was sorry I left home after such a row,' cried a
daughter at her mother's funeral.

One moment you're weeping on each other's shoulders and
the next stunned by childish rivalries and resentments. 'Daddy
always loved my brother best.' 'She can't wait to get her hands
on the Chippendale dining table and chairs.'

Grief destroys concentration and induces a numbing inertia.
When my father died, it was months before I could sit before

my word processor with any kind of enthusiasm. Only the most uncerebral physical tasks would tempt me into action. 'No one ever told me about the laziness of grief,' wrote C.S. Lewis in *A Grief Observed*. '. . . I loathe the slightest effort. Not only writing but even reading a letter is too much.'

Hard as it is to believe at the time, a day will come when you wake up and everything is possible again. The haunting, harrowing memories of death and dying are replaced by older, happier ones, full of life and vigour. Not that you ever 'get over' a bereavement. The pain will diminish, gradually and with sudden heart-stopping waves of sorrow, but the loss you carry within you forever.

How to cope? Once again the best advice is 'don't bottle it up'. The more you talk the better. Talk about everything – your regrets, anger, love, irritation, your own fear of death and of being alone. Not just once but over and over. Talk to one person in the morning, and another in the evening and then start all over again.

Don't be afraid to cry. 'Some little thing would start me weeping,' said Ruth, whose mother had died six months before. 'Nothing to do with Mum at first; I'd be tired, the kids would get on top of me, the car wouldn't go or Alan would be late from work. I'd start crying and not be able to stop. Terrible storms of tears that tore me up until I was exhausted and maybe fell asleep. And afterwards I'd feel strangely healed and full of energy.'

References

CRUSE (an organisation for all those who have suffered a bereavement which offers advice, counselling and helpful publications)
   Cruse House,
   126 Sheen Road,
   Richmond,
   Surrey TW9 1UR
   (tel. 081-940 4818)

Cruse counselling line (9.30a.m. – 5p.m., Mon–Fri) 081-332 7227

Living With Grief by Dr Tony Lake (Sheldon)

LONELINESS

We need others. Scientists have shown that in lonely people, those who find it difficult to make friends, or who are isolated for one reason or another, the number of natural killer cells in the immune system is depleted, leaving them more susceptible to viral infections of every kind. Companionship, sharing jokes and confidences, on the other hand, prompts the release of endorphins, the brain chemicals associated with pleasure.

Lonely is not the same as alone. There are individuals, usually introverts whose sense of self comes from within rather than those around them, who are content to spend hours, even days, on their own. Like dolphins surfacing for air, they'll take their socialising as and when they require it.

But the truly lonely are trapped. They might be young mothers with small children, living alone in urban tower blocks, or in sleepy suburbs hundreds of miles from their parents and friends. They might be awkward young students away from home for the first time, eating solitary meals in seedy flats and bedsitting rooms, too frightened of rejection, or ridicule, to reach out and make contact with others. They could be the old woman living next door; the widower in the flat above; the divorcee at the end of the street. They could be you.

For all kinds of peculiar reasons, people can build up barriers between themselves and others. They resist making approaches because one person might look boring, or superior, or another comes from a different culture, or class, or generation.

Their own self-esteem is so low, and their social skills so inadequate, that meeting people is terrifying. Nobody will speak to them. They'll say the wrong thing. Be ignored.

Laughed at. 'I'm too shy,' they'll mutter apologetically. 'No one's interested in me.' But shyness is too often a mask for monumental self-centredness.

Lonely people are rarely energetic people. They're eaten up with inner tension that drains their zest and they become lethargic. Nothing is worth doing.

It's a gritty fact of life that the only person who can help you overcome your loneliness is yourself. The chances are minimal that somebody will suddenly look up and say 'Wow, there's Ben. Even though he won't open his mouth and hangs in the corner, I can just tell that underneath lurks a sparkling conversationalist with a rapier wit.'

This is hard. It means learning social skills, like actually looking at other people instead of at their toes, listening to them, taking an interest in what they're saying, asking them about themselves, seeing things from another person's point of view. It means not being ultra sensitive and taking offence easily. It means accepting generosity with grace. It means sharing your own thoughts and feelings, being ready to laugh at yourself, and yes, maybe doing people the honour of trusting them with your vulnerability.

BOREDOM

Boredom? Yes, boredom. Being bored because you don't have enough to do is as stressful as having too much to cope with. Far from being overstretched, your resources are not sufficiently stimulated to keep them fit and active. Adrenalin levels twice as high as normal have been discovered in people doing boring work; the frustration puts them under excessive stress.

Who is bored? Adolescents who have not learnt the skill of concentration complain most commonly of boredom. These may be the ones who, in search of excitement, steal cars and beat up innocent people going about their business.

Up to 56 per cent of British employees say their entire job is boring; 87 per cent report feeling bored sometimes. The boredom of long-distance lorry drivers and airline pilots who fall asleep at the wheel and the cockpit could be responsible for motorway pile-ups and air crashes. 'The job is 99 per cent sheer tedium and 1 per cent terror,' remarked the captain of a jumbo jet. With eleven hours of night flying and the plane on automatic pilot, one can see why.

Boredom researchers suggest allotting less time to boring tasks – something most of us unconsciously do already. Another technique is called 'stimulation management', or using the imagination to keep you alert. Think of those interminable car games you play with the children: I-spy, counting white vans, and turning number plates into anagrams.

If you're bored because you haven't got a job, or the one you have doesn't occupy enough of your time, then find something to do. Take up voluntary work or a hobby. Join a class at your local adult education college. These suggestions may seem screamingly obvious, but you would be astonished at how many people sit about moaning on the one hand that they're bored, and on the other that they're too tired to make a move.

ANXIETY AND PANIC ATTACKS

The physical symptoms alone of anxiety are exhausting: shortness of breath, dizziness, a pounding heart, trembling, muscle tension, sweating, numbness, dry mouth, stomach aches and nausea. The full force of the 'fight or flight' response to danger is turned on by a single fearful thought.

Helen was terrified of being enclosed in small spaces from which she couldn't escape; a fear known as claustrophobia. Riding in lifts, for instance, was almost impossible for her. What if it stopped between floors? They might be stuck for hours and she couldn't get out. Perhaps the wires would snap and it would plummet down the lift well, dashing them all to their deaths.

Helen tried to disguise her anxiety. It hadn't quite reached a stage where she refused point blank to get into an elevator, but if there was no alternative she would enter it with the dread of a French aristocrat facing the guillotine. Her eyes were fixed on the floor indicator, her hands were clammy and her heart raced. As soon as the doors opened, she bolted out. It was an agonising experience, and so she adopted a classic form of coping behaviour.

She avoided lifts whenever possible, sometimes climbing stairs to the fifth or sixth floor. 'I need more exercise,' she explained as she headed for the staircase. She turned down the opportunity of at least one job because it would mean working on the twenty-fifth floor of a building and taking the lift several times a day.

Even so, her anxiety was not as crippling as that of a fully fledged agoraphobic, someone who panics at the thought of stepping outside their house. It's estimated that nine million Britons will suffer from abnormal anxiety at some time. This utterly debilitating state of tension includes phobias and panic attacks; a sudden onset of frightening symptoms – heart palpitations, dizziness, difficulty in breathing, and faintness – that are so unpleasant the sufferer will do anything to avoid them again. They become afraid of fear.

Those most prone to such terrors tend to be highly strung and over-sensitive individuals, often with overheated imaginations to match. If you're born with a tendency to anxiety, or brought up with anxious parents, it could take only fifteen minutes stuck on the Underground between stations to prompt a panic attack. The next time you step on the tube or it slows unexpectedly, you anticipate another attack. Finally you don't take the Underground at all. A traumatic event, a bad bout of flu, or a long period of stress can also tip the balance.

Alice Neville battled against her own panic attacks and believes that most sufferers can take steps to help themselves. She gives advice via an information service, PAX.

Self-help

★ Learn how to relax completely and breathe correctly (see Chapters 7 and 9) and do this at the first onset of panic.

★ Undergo a gradual exposure to the objects or situations of fear. Helen, for example, worked on the third floor of a building and one day, instead of using the stairs, took the lift. It was a short ride and the next day she was able to use it twice. By steadily increasing the number of times she used elevators and the number of floors in a ride, she managed to gain control over her phobia. Whenever she gets in a lift, however, she always checks her 'escape route' – the position of the alarm, emergency stop and internal telephone if there is one. Alice, too, always made sure she had enough money for a taxi should a panic attack strike her in the street. Just knowing it was there helped her to behave normally.

★ Take a more positive attitude to life. Instead of imagining the worst, picture yourself coping with the situation you dread. Sailing with ease up to the forty-second floor of a skyscraper. Shopping happily in the supermarket. Stepping confidently aboard an aeroplane.

★ Distract yourself. Caroline suffered from panic attacks on buses and trains. When she felt the familiar symptoms, she filled her mind with a running monologue: 'I wonder where that woman is going with such a large bunch of roses, why red roses, is she meeting a friend, or perhaps her mother, or has a lover given them to her . . .?'

References

PAX – send s.a.e. to 4 Manor Brook,
   Blackheath,
   London SE3 9AW

Coping With Anxiety, tape produced by the Council for Involuntary Tranquilliser Addiction (CITA),
   Anxiety Tape,

PO Box 1,
Wirral L47 7DD
(£6.75 incl. p & p)

Panic Attacks by Christine Ingham (Thorsons)
Who's Afraid? by Alice Neville (Arrow)

COMPULSIONS AND OBSESSIONS

You wash your hands a hundred times a day to avoid contamination, or take three-quarters of an hour to leave the house because you have to check the iron is off, and the stove is off, and the washing machine and dryer and all the electrical appliances, not just once but forty and fifty times. As you can imagine, it is very tiring indeed.

In severe cases, it is best to get psychological help. Otherwise, if it takes you only five or ten minutes to get out the front door, try to cut down on the number of checks you make by leaving a longer interval between each one. Or postpone washing your hands for as long as possible. Picture the very worst that could happen (the house burns down, yes, because you left the iron on, but *you* weren't inside, were you?). In his book Dr Frank Tallis of the Institute of Psychiatry offers specific self-help strategies.

Reference

Understanding Obsessions and Compulsions by Dr Frank Tallis (Sheldon Press)

WORRY

Everyone worries. Some more than others, perhaps, but on the whole worry is part of the human condition. Will I finish that report in time for the meeting next week? Do we have enough money for a holiday? Will our son pass his exams? What is that lump on my back? Could it be cancer?

Unlike anxiety, which tends to be generalised – something dreadful will happen if I step outside the door, my heart will burst, I'll feel sick and faint – worry is usually specific. There *are* chronic worriers, who solve one worry and look around for another as a way of masking underlying anxiety, but on the whole, worry can actually be good for you.

It's a kind of internal alarm system that nags at you until you deal with a problem, and gives you a chance to practise various strategies. If you're lying awake worrying why your teenage daughter hasn't come home, you've probably rehearsed the accident-hospital-police scenario. Which is why you jump down her throat when she tiptoes in forty-five minutes past the allotted hour.

Accomplished worriers seem to be slower at making decisions, say psychologists, possibly because their parents had high expectations of them and disapproved of mistakes, so they strive very hard to make sure a decision is 'right'. The snag, of course, is that more often than not you will never have enough information to be 100 per cent sure of being 'right', and the longer you fuss, the worse the worry becomes.

Get your worrying in perspective. Whether you'll catch the train to Bristol in time is peanuts compared to the worries confronting Elizabeth, whose husband died of a long illness leaving her with financial problems, two small children and a house in a state of decay. 'How do you cope when things are very bad?' she says. 'You keep a sense of humour. When Roger was sick we switched off the gloomy TV programmes and watched the funny ones. You talk to generous-minded friends. You think "what is the worst possible thing that can happen, and can I do anything about it?" and if not, you leave it.'

Self-help

★ Make a list of your worries. Tackle those that can be dealt with (go to the doctor about any lumps), and put the rest aside until you're able to think about them clearly. Allow yourself half an hour's worry time a day so that you expend less energy on fruitless agitation.

★ Identify the worry. The friction between you and your colleague at the office may be only a reflection of the real problem – the fact that you want to change jobs.

★ Brainstorm solutions. Write down even the daftest suggestions, such as 'rob a bank' or 'disappear up the Amazon'. This way you'll have more of a choice.

★ Replace negative thoughts with realistic ones. I was fretting over our 17-year-old son taking his sister's car to go to the Glastonbury pop festival with two friends. 'Will he have enough money? What if it rains? What if they have an accident? Where will they sleep?' 'But they'll love it,' said my friend Sylvia. 'What fun for them all, and so good for them to be independent for a couple of days.' And immediately the scene shifted in my mind, and the sun, as it were, came out. Of course it would be fun, they were sensible boys and it was time I stopped fussing over him.

★ Talk to friends. 'A worry shared is a worry halved.'

★ Accept there are some problems that you can do nothing about.

★ If a worry won't go away, try changing your response. Learn to ignore it, or, painful as it might be, face up to it.

★ Don't squander energy worrying about what might happen. Your daughter *might* fail her exams. You *might* fall under a bus. The plane *might* be delayed; you *might* miss your connection. In the meantime, there's absolutely nothing you can do about it.

'We think the ideal life is stress-free,' says Elizabeth, 'and it's not, and we shouldn't expect it to be. The more you realise trials are part of life and welcome them as challenges, the more you can stop wasting energy and enjoy living.'

Reference

How to Stop Worrying by Dr Frank Tallis (Sheldon Press)

SEEKING HELP

Modern society gallops at such a heedless pace that those we traditionally turned to for emotional support – priests, family doctors, wise old relatives and neighbours – are no longer available. They're too busy, they live too far away, they're never in.

Talking to a psychologist or a counsellor is no longer seen as a sign of gibbering insanity, but simply a means of coping. Thousands of people do it every day.

When should I ask for help?

Situations when you feel so overwhelmed you can't cope can usually be blamed on one or more of what therapists call the 'three Cs'.

★ **Choice:** You can't decide what step to take next. Should you leave your partner? Should you take a new job? You simply don't know what to do for the best.

★ **Change:** Marriage, parenthood, mid-life, divorce, retirement, bereavement – moving from one life stage to another can be traumatic.

★ **Confusion:** You can't understand why you feel distressed, but your suffering has taken over your life and you can't control it.

How will I find help?

First port of call should be your GP. Psychotherapy and counselling are available free on the NHS, but some areas are better served than others, and you may have to do your own chasing. The alternative of course is to pay, which could set you back £30 per session on average.

Be as clear as possible in advance about what kind of therapy you want. 'Do you want it to be a "cool" or a "warm" place?' suggests Brigid, a counsellor. 'Do you want to work more on your feelings or on your thinking and behaviour? Would you prefer the therapist to be in charge, or do you need to be in control? Or do you like an equal relationship?'

Counselling tends to focus on a specific problem and treatment is seen in terms of weeks, not months or even years. A counsellor is skilled in listening and prompting, and will be supportive ('warm') but give little or no direct advice. You'll be encouraged to draw on your own resources for insight into your problems.

Psychotherapy helps you examine past experiences and relationships to deal with deep-seated personal issues – why you are as you are – that can bring profound changes. One therapist compares it to disentangling a knot: 'You loosen a bit, and some unravels, and then you work at another piece until that is freed, and finally everything is released.'

Psychoanalysts, like psychotherapists, take you back through childhood to unearth memories and emotions buried in the unconscious. It's a long and frequently expensive process, and in order to encourage you to transfer any feelings you have about people onto the analyst, he or she will reveal little about themselves ('cool').

Psychologists have taken a university degree. **Clinical psychologists** work in many areas of the NHS, where treatment for complaints such as phobias often involves behavioural therapy – training people to deal with problems by changing their behaviour. For example, rather than exploring *why* you hate spiders, you'll be gradually exposed to them until you lose your fear.

Psychiatrists initially train as doctors and then specialise in mental disorders, such as schizophrenia or depression. They tend to treat patients primarily with drugs, although many offer or refer you to psychotherapy as well.

It's a scandalous fact that anyone can do a weekend course and stick up a plate calling themselves a psychotherapist. Protect yourself by making sure that your counsellor or psychotherapist is registered with the British Association for Counselling (BAC) or the UK Standing Conference for Psychotherapy.

The BAC has a resources directory listing counselling and

psychotherapy centres as well as individual practitioners in private practice. It also publishes an excellent booklet *Is It For Me?*

References

British Association for Counselling,
  1 Regent Place,
  Rugby,
  Warwickshire CV21 2PJ
  (tel. 0788 578328)

British Association of Psychotherapists,
  37 Mapesbury Road,
  London NW2
  (tel. 081-452 9823)

Institute of Family Therapy,
  43 New Cavendish Street,
  London W1M 7RG
  (tel. 071-935 1651)

Institute of Group Analysis,
  1 Daleham Gardens,
  London NW3 5BY
  (tel. 071-431 2693)

Metanoia Psychotherapy Training Institute,
  (humanistic and transpersonal ['warm'] therapies emphasising the whole person),
  13 North Common Road,
  London W5 2QB
  (tel. 081-579 2505)

Psychosynthesis and Education Trust,
  48 Guildford Road,
  London SW8 2BU

(tel. 071-622 8295)
(transpersonal therapy)

Tavistock Clinic,
   120 Belsize Lane,
   London NW3 5BA
   (tel. 071-435 7111)

UK Standing Conference for Psychotherapy,
   167 Sumatra Road,
   London NW6 1PN
   (tel. 071-431 4379)

Westminster Pastoral Foundation,
   23 Kensington Square,
   London W8 5HN
   (tel. 071-937 6956)
   (highly regarded Government-subsidised therapy)

The Women's Therapy Centre,
   6-9 Manor Gardens,
   London N7 6LA
   (tel. 071-263 6200)
   (psychoanalytic and group therapy)

Families and how to survive them by Robin Skynner and John
   Cleese (Mandarin)
Life and how to survive it by Robin Skynner and John Cleese
   (Methuen)

CHAPTER 14

Last but not least

THE SPIRIT IS WILLING

Tired in body, tired in mind. But what about the spirit? We forget, so easily, that very essence of ourselves. Sometimes we don't even know how to find it. And yet weariness of spirit lies at the heart of so much of our tiredness.

What *is* the spirit? Everything. Anything. Our soul, the Self, the anima. That which makes us peculiarly, individually you or I, over and above the network of muscle and bone and nerve, the cascades of hormones and chemicals. What drives you, inspires you, moves you.

So how do we go about restoring it? The answer – beyond the scope of this book – is for each of us to discover for ourselves. But begin by thinking about those things that are deeply important to you. Remember some of the pleasures you might have listed, back in Chapter 10.

Creativity is one route. 'When I ignored my music,' said Alison, 'I cut off a part of me that I discovered was necessary for me to function as a whole. I can lose myself in making music on my violin, and come back to earth almost magically refreshed.'

Others have spoken of an energising 'high' when they are absorbed in creative work, writing or painting, even gardening and needlework. A kind of alert contentment that knits physical, mental and emotional aspects of yourself together, and which in itself is a source of power.

'I hadn't picked up my crayons and drawn for years,' said Janie. 'Then one day when I was very low and under a lot of pressure, I took them out and just let whatever was in my head come out. At first there was anger – all black and red and bold lines – and then the pictures became calmer, blues and greens, and sweeping shapes, and as they did so, so did I. It was wonderful.'

In a recent study in the US, when people took pen and paper and wrote for twenty minutes a day about the pain and frustration they felt at being made redundant, they were more likely to be successful in finding another job – an indication that they were presenting themselves more positively – than those who had bottled up their feelings.

Listening to music, looking at pictures or reading poetry doesn't release quite the same wellsprings of energy, but it is a soothing, stroking experience that takes you out of yourself. Compare tastes with your friends: ask them what music they like to hear when they're tired and want to feel better. Watching television doesn't count; we view it too uncritically, a gooey marshmallow for the senses, so that the inner, perceptive you goes to sleep.

More and more research shows that our states of mind are inextricably connected with our physical responses. In one study, listening to Bach induced brain wavelengths similar to those of meditation.

Laugh as much as you can. It will prompt biochemical changes in the brain, releasing a wave of energy-giving adrenalin and endorphins into the bloodstream. Laughter, doctors are discovering, is an antidote to stress, reducing blood pressure and muscle tension, deepening breathing and improving circulation. In Birmingham, stress counsellor Robert Holden runs an NHS laughter therapy clinic, whose clients include overwrought doctors who have forgotten how to smile.

Make the most of your friends. An extraordinary study at the University of California has demonstrated the power of emotional support groups: when a group of women with breast cancer met regularly to talk and share their feelings, they survived twice as long as women who lacked this companionship.

'I joined a reading group that opened up valued new friendships,' says Sarah, a secondary school teacher. 'There's about

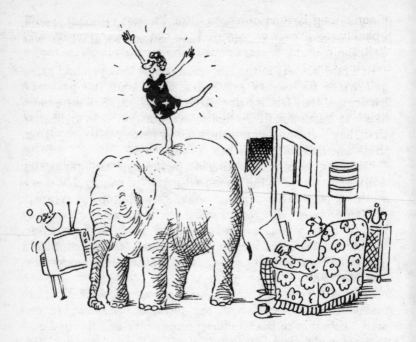

eight or ten of us and we meet once a month to discuss a particular book that we've read. We're all women, all very different – one is at home with children, another is a doctor – but we chew over all sorts of subjects, exchange ideas and attitudes way outside the structure of the meeting. We found we were *caring* about each other.'

Physically caring for others, when your time and efforts are freely given, has been so frequently associated with agreeable bodily sensations, and even the easing of ailments like headaches and depression, that it is known as the 'helper's high'. In one American survey, 88 per cent of people doing volunteer work described an identifiable feeling that one woman compared to the sense of fitness and well-being she felt while swimming. The old axiom that doing something nice for someone gives a warm glow is literally true.

There's no denying that 'spirit' implies an acknowledgement

of something beyond ourselves. But I'm not religious, you'll probably say. Never go to church, or synagogue, or whatever. Well, there are more ways of nourishing yourselves spiritually than kneeling in a pew.

Prayer *is* vital for some, and appears to have a remarkable power for those who believe in it, but take off your blinkers and step off the stress treadmill for a moment. Notice not just who you are, but where you are. Reach outside yourself. Becoming aware that you are a part of a wider context, whether it's the human race or the environment, seems to be an enlarging experience – and an enlivening one.

References

The Laughter Clinic,
  34 Denewood Avenue,
  Handsworth Wood,
  Birmingham B20 2AB
  (tel. 021-551 2932)

Recovering the Soul and *Meaning and Medicine* by Dr Larry
  Dossey (Bantam)

Index

Abbey, Dr Susan 186
Acupressure 96–7
Acupuncture 43–4
  for chronic pain 31–2
  for PMT 35
Aerobic exercise 131–2, 134–5
Air conditioning systems 65
Air ions 65–6
Alcohol 103, 124–5
Alexander Technique 31, 178–9
Allergies 14–18
  identifying 16–17
  treating symptoms 17
  wheat products 15, 16
All Hallows House 144
Alternative medicine
  choosing a therapist 41–3
  chronic pain and 31–2
  costs of treatment 41
  role of 40–43
  useful books and tapes 50–51
Amarant Trust 28, 30
Anaemia 18–21
  iron deficiency 18–19
  megaloblastic 19
  pernicious 19
  sickle-cell 20
  symptoms 18
  thalassemia 20
Antidepressants, new breed of
  189–90
Anxiety 196–9
Appearance, confidence in your
  160–61
Aromatherapy 44–5
  anaemia and 21
  baths with essential oils 95

benefits of 174–5
massage 96
oils for diabetics 25
for PMT 35
for Seasonal Affective Disease 75
Assertiveness training 155–70
Autogenic training 179–80

Bach flower remedies 41, 45–6
Back problems, office chairs 68–70
Badminton 136
Ball, Jillian 186
Basil 127
Bath, taking a
  bicarbonate of soda as additive 95
  as reliever of stress 95
Behavioural psychology 159
Bicarbonate of soda as bath additive
  95
Biofeedback 184
Boredom 195–6
Brain, influence of the, on physical
  health 89–90
Breathing, importance of correct
  139–41

Cabbage as provider of selenium 127
Caffeine 37, 103, 124–6
Calcium 121
Calman, Mel 187
Camomile tea 35
Cancer 21–2
Candida albicans 22–4
Carbohydrates 110
Cartesian Dualism 88
Celloids 123

Central heating 65
Chairs, back problems and 68–70
Change, The (Germaine Greer) 28
Chiropractic 46
Chronic fatigue syndrome 1–11; *see also* Myalgic encephalitis (ME)
Churchill, Winston 98, 187
Clare, Dr Anthony 188, 189
Clinical psychologists 203
Colour therapy 180–81
Communication between working mums and husbands 167–70
Compulsions 199
Confidence building 155–70
Contraceptive pill 37
Counselling 203
CRUSE 193–4
Cycling 135

Dancing 135
Davies, Philippa 160
Depression 185–92
    causes of 188–90
    checklist for 188
    self-help 190–91
Detoxification diets 124
Diabetes 24–6
Dickson, Anne 150, 162, 163
Diet
    bad eating 108
    breakfast 126
    carbohydrates 110
    conflicting advice 109
    detoxification 124
    diabetic 25
    energy foods 127
    fats 114, 126
    food supplements 109
    fruit and vegetable 112–13
    hypoglycaemia 25–6
    insomnia 103
    iron deficiency and 20
    menopausal 30
    mood-changing foods 124–6
    for PMT 34
    protein 113–14
    rules for a healthy 109–10
    for Seasonal Affective Disease 75
    starchy foods, importance 110

sugars 110–12
for thrush 23–4
thyroid disorders and 36
vitamins, *see that title*
Doctors
    attitude to alternative medicine 41
    consulting your GP 12–14, 39–40, 202
Do-in 176
Drugs
    side-effects of 37
    useful books concerning 37–8
Dust mites 17

Emotions, influence on physical health 89–90
Environment, problems caused by the 64–75
Essential oils as bath additive 95
Evening primrose oil 34
Exercise
    aerobic 131–2, 134–5
    badminton 136
    breathing 140
    choosing type of 133–7
    cycling 135
    dancing 135
    energy booster 140
    maximum heart rate during 131
    meditation 183
    mind and body 137–9
    'moderate' and 'mindful' 130
    for muscle tension 94–5, 106–7
    pulse rate 132–3
    regular 128–41
    relaxation, at your desk 92
    running and jogging 135
    and Seasonal Affective Disease 75
    to aid self-knowledge 147–52
    skiing 135
    stress, relief of 103–4
    swimming 136
    T'ai Chi 138–9
    tennis 136
    walking 136–7
    yoga 137–8
Family responsibilities, working mums and 155–9
Fasting 124

Fats in the diet 114
Fitness, importance of 128–41
Flotation 177–8
Flower remedies, *see* Bach flower remedies
Folates 119–20
Food fads 122–4
Food intolerance/allergies 15–16, 17
Food supplements 122–4
Formaldehyde 66
Fraser, Antonia 26
Fruit in the diet 112–13

Garlic, and diabetes 25
Giampaolo, Lisbeth 130
Ginseng in honey 127
Gorman, Teresa 28
GP, *see* Doctor
Green theme in offices 71
Greer, Germaine 28
Greer, Dr Stephen 89
Grief 192–4
Guarana 127

Hatha yoga for diabetics 25
Hayfever 14, 17
Healing resources 171–84
Health farms 98
Heaton, Ros 161
Help, seeking 202–5
Herbal remedies for
  anaemia 21
  insomnia 103
Herbalism 46–7
Hochschild, Dr Arlie 4
Holmes, Dr Thomas 83–4
Homeopathic medicine 47–8
  anaemia 21
  British Homeopathic Association 48
  menopause 30
  oral thrush 23
  PMT 35
  thyroid disorders 37
Hormone Replacement Therapy (HRT) 30–31
Horne, Professor Jim 101

Household chores
  stress caused by 94
  working mums and 155–9
Humidifiers 65
Husbands, working mums and their 166–70
Hypnotherapy 48–9
Hypoglycaemia 25–6

Immune system
  allergies and the 15
  stress and the 87–8
Input (pain clinic) 32
Insomnia 48
  bedtime snacks 103
  dealing with 99–104
  see also Sleep
Iodine 121
Ionisers 66, 75
Iron
  body's need for 121
  deficiency 18–19
  diet to rectify deficiency 20

Job satisfaction 146–7
Jogging 135

Kobasa, Suzanne 147

Laughter Clinic, The 209
Lifestyle, looking at your 39–40
Light
  in the office environment 71–2
  Seasonal Affective Disorder 72–5
Lindenfield, Gael 149
Liver, vitamins and minerals in 127
Loneliness 194–5

McWhirter, Jane 10, 144–5
Manganese 120
Massage
  benefits of 96
  as healing tool 172–6
  for PMT 35
Maxwell-Hudson, Clare 94, 173
ME, *see* Myalgic encephalomyelitis
Medical reasons for fatigue 12–38
Meditation 181–4
Mehrabian, Albert 160

Menopause 26–30
Menstruation, iron deficiency caused by heavy periods 19
Milligan, Spike 187
Mind, influence of the, on physical illness 88–90
Minerals 35, 37, 120–22
    deficiency 116–17
    supplements 123–4
Mood-changing foods 124–6
Muscle tension, exercise to relieve 94–5, 106–7
Myalgic encephalomyelitis (ME) 52–63
    case histories 60–63
    checklist of symptoms 58–9
    getting to grips with 53–4
    as 'lifestyle' disease 54–7
    mystery of 52–3
    psychiatric view of 57–8
    viral source as cause of 54
Myrrh, in treatment of oral thrush 23

Napping, benefits of 98–9
Naturopathy 49–50, 124
Neville, Alice 197
Nicholson, Emma 159
'No', how to say 163
Noise pollution 66–7
Nutritional supplements 122–4

Obsessions 199
Office environment, pollution 65–72
Organisations concerned with
    acupuncture 44
    Alexander Technique 179
    allergies 18
    alternative medicine 42–3
    aromatherapy 45
    autogenic training 179–80
    back pain 70
    biofeedback 184
    chiropractic 46
    colour therapy 181
    counselling 204–5
    depression 191–2
    flotation 178
    grief 193–4
    herbalism 47
    homeopathy 48
    hypnotherapy 49
    marriage guidance 170
    massage 173, 174–5
    ME 63
    meditation 184
    the menopause 30
    naturopathy 50
    osteopathy 50
    pain 32–3, 70
    premenstrual tension 35–6
    psychotherapy 204–5
    reflexology 177
    Seasonal Affective Disease 75
    self-knowledge 154
    shiatsu 176
    sleep matters 103
    the spirit 209
    T'ai Chi 139
    yoga 138
Osteopathy 50
    useful books 50–51
Osteoporosis 28, 30
Overweight, dealing with 115–16

Pain
    acupuncture as aid 31–2
    chronic 30–33
    visualisation as aid 32
Pain Relief Foundation 32
Painkillers 31
Panic attacks 196–9
Patel, Dr Chandra 82
PAX 197, 198
Personality, effect of regular exercise on 129–30
Pert, Dr Candace 89, 90, 91
Phosphorus 121–2
Photocopiers, pollution from 66
Physical fitness, importance of 128–41
Pither, Dr Charles 32
Plants in the office environment 71
Potassium 122
Premenstrual Tension (PMT) 33–6
Protein in the diet 113–14
Psychiatrists 203

Psychoanalysts 203
Psychologists 203
Psychotherapy counselling 39–40, 203

Rahe, Dr Richard 83–4
Rantzen, Esther 151
Rapaport, Dr Mark 62, 186
Reflexology
  benefits of 176–7
  thyroid disorders 37
Relate 168, 170
Relaxation technique 104, 106–7
RelaxPlus programme 184
Remedies for relief of stress and
  tiredness 92–107
Rosemary 127
Rowe, Dr Dorothy 188
Royal Jelly 127
Running 135

Salt in the diet 120
Seasonal Affective Disorder (SAD)
  72–5
Selenium 121, 127
Self-help
  allergies 16–17
  anaemia 20–21
  anxiety and panic attacks 198–9
  chronic pain 32–3
  depression 190–91
  diabetes 25
  menopause 28–30
  premenstrual tension 34–6
  stress 90–91
  thrush 23–4
  worry 200–201
Self-knowledge 142–54
  case history 142–4
  exercises to aid 147–53
Sesame seeds 127
Sex, the menopause and 29
Sheehy, Gail 26, 27
Shiatsu 175–6
Ship (Self-Help Pain Management)
  32, 33
Shower, as pick-me-up to relieve
  stress 95

Sick Building Syndrome 64–5
Skiing 135
Skin brush 96
Sleep
  achieving a good night 99–104
  categories of sleeplessness 102
  drop-off tips 103–4
  individual requirements 101
  patterns of 99–100
  perceptions of 101
  sleep restriction therapy 102
  sleeping pills 102
  see also Insomnia
Smoking, insomnia and 103
Sodium 120
Space control in offices 70
Spirit, restoring the 206–9
'Springboard' development
  programme 150, 153, 160
Steptoe, Professor Andrew 87
Stress
  case histories 77–9, 86
  causes of 8–11, 84–7
  checklist on how well you cope 105
  dealing with stressors 77
  effect on immune system 87–8
  emotional signs of 83
  failure to recognise symptoms 81–2
  fatigue as symptom of 6–11, 76–7
  'fight or flight' response 80
  household chores as source of 94
  lower levels in fit people 129
  mind–body connection 87–91
  physical symptoms of chronic 82–3
  visualisation exercise 92–3
  walking as relief for 94
Sugar in the diet 110–12
Sunflower seeds 127
Sunlight, Seasonal Affective Disease
  72–5
Swimming 136

T'ai-chi Ch'uan (T'ai Chi) 138–9
Tallis, Dr Frank 199
Tanner, Susan 186
Tea, and iron absorption 121
Technology, tyranny of 4–6
Tennis 136
Thatcher, Margaret 101

Thrush 22–4
  diet 23–4
  oral 23
  symptoms 22
  vaginal 23
Thyroid disorders 36–7
Time
  controlling your 164–8
  sharing 166–8
Tired All the Time Syndrome (TATT)
  1–11
Tissue salts 123
Turner, Julie 87

Vacuuming, allergies and 17
VDUs, mental and physical fatigue
  from 67–8
Vegetables in the diet 112–13
Visualisation 32
  as aid to sleep 104
  as reliever of stress 92–3
Vitamins 34–5, 36–7, 75, 117–19
  deficiency 116–17

  supplements 123
Voice, projecting your 160

Walking 94, 136–7
Ware, Norma 55, 56, 57
Weekend break, taking a 97
Willis, Liz 150, 160
Winter blues 74–5
Working environment, pollution in
  the 65–72
Working mums
  fatigue suffered by 2–6
  household chores 3–4
  husbands of 166–70
  problems of 155–9
  sleep patterns of 4
  time management 164–70
Worry 199–201

Yoga 137–8
Yoghurt in treatment of thrush 23

Zinc 121

Headline Health Kicks

Positive and practical advice to relieve persistent health problems.
Titles available include:

THE PRIME OF YOUR LIFE
Self help during menopause   Pamela Armstrong   £5.99 ☐

STOP COUNTING SHEEP
Self help for insomnia sufferers   Dr Paul Clayton   £5.99 ☐

AM I A MONSTER, OR IS THIS PMS?
Self help for PMS sufferers   Louise Roddon   £5.99 ☐

GET UP AND GO!
Self help for fatigue sufferers   Anne Woodham   £5.99 ☐

You can kick that problem!

All Headline books are available at your local bookshop or newsagent, or can be ordered direct from the publisher. Just tick the titles you want and fill in the form below. Prices and availability subject to change without notice.

Headline Book Publishing Ltd, Cash Sales Department, Bookpoint, 39 Milton Park, Abingdon, OXON, OX14 4TD, UK. If you have a credit card you may order by telephone – 0235 831700.

Please enclose a cheque or postal order made payable to Bookpoint Ltd to the value of the cover price and allow the following for postage and packing:

UK & BFPO: £1.00 for the first book, 50p for the second book and 30p for each additional book ordered up to a maximum charge of £3.00.

OVERSEAS & EIRE: £2.00 for the first book, £1.00 for the second book and 50p for each additional book.

Name...

Address...

....

....

If you would prefer to pay by credit card, please complete:
Please debit my Visa/Access/Diner's Card/American Express (delete as applicable) card no:

Signature..   Expiry date...................